MENTAL REHEARSAL FOR WARRIORS

OTHER BOOKS BY LOREN W. CHRISTENSEN

The following are available on Amazon, from their publishers, and through the usual book outlets. Some are available as ebooks. Signed copies can be purchased at LWC Books, www.lwcbooks.com

Nonfiction

Street Stoppers
Fighting In The Clinch
Fighter's Fact Book
Fighter's Fact Book 2
Solo Training
Solo Training 2
Speed Training
The Fighter's Body
Total Defense
The Mental Edge
The Way Alone
Far Beyond Defensive Tactics
Fighting Power
Crouching Tiger
Anything Goes
Winning With American Kata
Total Defense
Riot
Warriors
On Combat
Warrior Mindset
Deadly Force Encounters
Surviving Workplace Violence
Surviving A School Shooting
Gangbangers
Skinhead Street Gangs
Hookers, Tricks And Cops
Way Of The Warrior
Skid Row Beat
Defensive Tactics
Missing Children
Fight Back: Self-Defense For Women
Extreme Joint Locking
Timing In The Martial Arts
Fighter's Guide to Hard-Core Heavy Bag Training
The Brutal Art Of Ripping, Poking And Pressing Vital Targets
How To Live Safely In A Dangerous World
Fighting The Pain Resistant Attacker
Evolution of Weaponry
Meditation for Warriors

Fiction

Dukkha: The Suffering
Dukkha: Reverb
Dukkha: Unloaded

MENTAL REHEARSAL FOR WARRIORS

For Cops, Soldiers, and Martial Artists

LOREN W. CHRISTENSEN

LWC Books

Copyright © 2014 Loren W. Christensen

All rights reserved.

No part of this book may be reproduced in any form or without written permission from the author.

For permissions, more information, or to reach the author, contact:

LWC BOOKS
PO Box 20311
Portland, Oregon
97294-0311
lwcbooks.com
sales@lwcbooks.com

Cover and Interior Design by Kamila Z. Miller
Background for the cover by Sirius-sdz
 http://sirius-sdz.deviantart.com/

ISBN-13: 978-1499779875
ISBN-10: 1499779879

Neither the author nor the publisher assumes any responsibility for the use or misuse of this book.

ACKNOWLEDGEMENTS

As always, much love to my wife Lisa Christensen for her support and patience when I'm writing, and all the other times too.

Thanks to the many people who have helped me with my meditation and mental rehearsal practice over the years.

Thanks to the cops, soldiers, and martial artists who told me of their mental rehearsal practices.

Thanks to Afghanistan war veteran and martial artist Kevin Faulk for his eagle eye at spotting errors in the manuscript.

CONTENTS

SECTION 1

Introduction	5
Chapter 1: Myths About Mental Rehearsal	11
Chapter 2: Why Warriors Need to Practice Mental Rehearsal	15
Chapter 3: Nuts And Bolts About Meditation	19

SECTION 2

Chapter 4: Introduction to Meditation Methods	35
Chapter 5: Meditation Techniques	39
Chapter 6: 60-Second Meditations	67

SECTION 3

Chapter 7: Introduction To Mental Rehearsal	75
Chapter 8: Nuts And Bolts of Mental Rehearsal	79
Chapter 9: Mental Rehearsal Methods	85
Chapter 10: Mental Rehearsal Without Meditation	139
Bonus: Chapter 11: Mental Rehearsal For School Teachers	143
Conclusion	147
About the Author	149

HOW TO READ THIS BOOK

You will benefit the most by reading this book from beginning to end, in that order. While that might sound logical to some, it isn't always for people like me. I read magazines from back to front and when reading books like this one, I like to jump right to the techniques. If you're a "jumper," don't do that because you will miss a lot of small tips throughout the book (I think of them as golden nuggets) that make the various meditation methods and mental imagery techniques even more effective. For example, a tip noted in one technique will also be helpful in earlier ones as well as later ones.

Many meditation and mental rehearsal methods contain similar structures and verbiage. This was done on purpose so you can later jump to a technique and proceed without having to reference earlier how-to-do-it chapters.

For ease of writing and reading, the word(s):

"Soldiers" denotes the brave men and women in all military branches.

"Cops" and "police" denote the brave men and women in all law enforcement agencies.

"Martial artists" denotes the hard training men and women in all styles and systems.

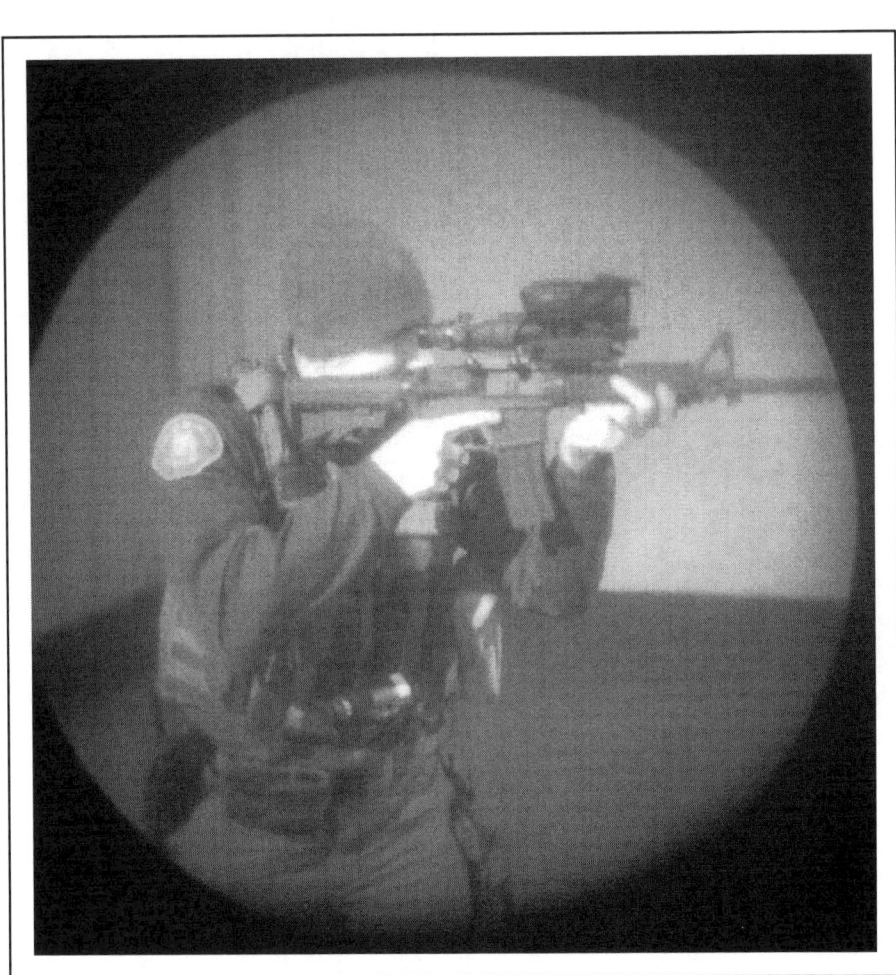

SECTION 1

Introduction
Chapter 1: Myths About Mental Rehearsal
Chapter 2: Why Warriors Need to Practice Mental Rehearsal
Chapter 3: Nuts And Bolts About Meditation

"I have a system of ridding my mind of negative thoughts. I visualize myself writing them down on a piece of paper. Then I imagine myself crumpling up the paper, lighting it on fire, and burning it to a crisp."

~ Bruce Lee

"Imagery exercises not only [should] be incorporated into "regular" police training and practice but officers [should] use mental imagery whenever they have a spare moment to improve their performance in what may be life-or-death situations."

~ Researchers, Netherlands

"I had a clear vision of myself winning the Mr. Universe contest. It was a very spiritual thing, in a way, because I had such faith in the route, the path, that there was never a question in my mind that I would make it."

~ Arnold Schwarzenegger

"There is no right or wrong way to meditate. Anyone who says otherwise is ignorant, a liar, or has some other agenda."

~ Anon

INTRODUCTION

Mental rehearsal, sometimes called mental imagery or visualization, is a natural process and one of the most powerful psychological tools to improve your warrior skills, be it in law enforcement, military, or martial arts. Actually, you already use mental rehearsal to some degree when you think about engaging in one of your warrior activities, such as raiding a drug house, engaging the enemy on some dusty foreign street, or facing an opponent in the ring.

Not long ago, mental rehearsal was commonly called "visualization," a term that limited the process to only one of your five senses. As you shall see shortly, mental rehearsal involves *all* of your senses to totally engage your mind and body in this incredible process.

Some 90 percent of athletes and 94 percent of coaches surveyed at the US Olympic Training Center said they used mental rehearsal. Of those, 97 percent of the athletes and 100 percent of the coaches agreed it improved their performance in their events. Keep in mind these are our top athletes. They don't waste time on anything that doesn't work.

Chuck Norris

As noted above, mental rehearsal used to be called visualization. The first time I heard the term was at a Chuck Norris seminar back in the '80s. He said he would go off and sit somewhere before his fight and visualize what was going to happen in his match. If he knew his opponent and his specialties, he would "see" in his mind's eye the fighter's kick and punch. Then Norris would visualize his own response to the attack: his block or avoidance and his successful counterattack to garner a point.

He would visualize this so intensely and so clearly, there was no doubt in Norris's mind that it would happen. He would even visualize himself raising his hand in victory and accepting the big trophy. His win was so crystal clear in his mind that on those rare occasions when he didn't win, it surprised him.

You have to wonder if Chuck Norris had used all five of his senses in his mental rehearsal, as you will learn here, how much better he would have done.

Speaking of athletes

Swimmer Michael Phelps used mental rehearsal and relaxation techniques before his Summer Olympics races. Phil Jackson, head coach of the Los Angeles Lakers, encourages his players to image victory before games. Tiger Woods, golf champion of the Earth, uses mental rehearsal as part of his practice routine.

Definitions

A quick search online reveals several definitions of mental rehearsal that are either inaccurate or limiting. For example, some say mental rehearsal is:

- seeing in your mind's eye.
- having a picture in your head.
- forming mental images.
- picturing mental images.
- having/seeing a mental image/picture.
- forming mental images of tasks or events.
- visualizing mental images.

These aren't wrong but they are incomplete. In this text you not only engage your mind's eye to see, but also learn how to feel, smell, hear, and even taste your mentally rehearsed image to make it as real as you possibly can.

Some might ask, "But didn't you call it mental imagery in *Meditation For Warriors*?" Dang, you caught me. Yes, I did. But after thinking and writing on the subject more, and talking with others in the warrior community, I believe "mental rehearsal" is a more fitting term. Plus it takes the mysticism out of it.

With this in mind, let's make our definition this:

Mental rehearsal is a way to use your imagination to improve your warrior skills.

Sweatless practice

I've written a few articles for magazines on mental imagery in which I called it "sweatless practice." Yes, thank you. I think it's clever too.

The name fits because you can do it sitting in the shade of a tree, in your easy chair, in a squad car during a stakeout, while on the way to a high-risk mission, and while waiting to compete in a martial arts sports competition. You don't need to stretch and warm up to do it, you don't need to wear special clothes (you can do it in the bathtub), nor do you need to perform any kind of ritual or formality.

All you need to do is close your eyes and experience your activity in your head. That said, while it's often preferred to do it with your eyes closed, you will learn ways to do it with them open so as not to draw attention to yourself.

In *Warrior Mindset*, a book I co-wrote with Dr. Mike Askens and Lt. Col. Dave Grossman, we used the term "Tactical Performance Imagery." Mental rehearsal is that, but I think the word "tactical" is becoming overused these days. So let's stick with mental rehearsal.

It's not woo-woo

I've been training and teaching the martial arts for self-defense since 1965. I've always emphasized that hand-to-hand combat must be simplistic. A physical confrontation is often explosive and violent and, as such, there is no place for over-the-top techniques that are better served in the movies than in the harsh reality of true violence.

I have also taken this no frills approach to meditation and to mental rehearsal. As with the martial arts, I strive to trim what is unnecessary and emphasize what is left. To my mind, why would you do otherwise?

In my Introduction to *Meditation for Warriors*, I made it clear the material as presented isn't hippy-dippy, crystal rubbing, incense burning, or goat sacrificing, all the things I classify as woo-woo. Such is the case with mental rehearsal.

There are people who want to make anything to do with the mind mystical, supernatural and, well, woo-woo. We wish these people well (while keeping our goats locked up) and if they want to dance in a sunset and bow to volcanoes, fine. But as a member of the warrior community, you want to keep things simple but productive.

Who is the bald-headed guy writing this?

I'm not an old hippy or a new ager, or a vegetarian, although I grew up in the hippy era, I like new age music, and love some vegetarian dishes. I began training in the martial arts in 1965, went into the Army in 1967, did a tour in Vietnam, joined the Portland Police Bureau in Oregon in 1972, and retired 25 years later. I've written lots of books on the fighting arts, books on an assortment of subcultures, others on preparing for and surviving the aftermath of violence and, of late, a police-thriller fiction series called *Dukkha*.

While researching a martial arts book in 1989, I became interested in the incredible power of incorporating the mind into my training. I had already been practicing mental rehearsal (I called it visualization at the time) and later discovered self-hypnosis, which some hypnotists admit is basically meditation with suggestions.

With the help of some teachers from diverse backgrounds, I quickly discovered the incredible power of meditation and mental rehearsal. Over the years since, I've learned meditation from writers, but mostly from various sifu and sensei while meditating in Zen monasteries, and other temples.

Here are two things I learned early on about meditation and mental rehearsal:

- It's incredibly simple.
- Too many people want to make it complicated and mystical.

I'm not a cave-dwelling sage and I don't wear a gold robe. I'm just a guy who has survived a warrior lifestyle who now passes on what I've learned.

Mental rehearsal is easy to do

How can I claim this since I don't know you? Because I know you already do it. But unless you've trained to do it formally, your mental rehearsal has probably been a tad unstructured and a little haphazard. No problem; it's an easy fix.

Let's say:

- Your sergeant tells you that after chow you're going to get refresher training on IED (improvised explosive device) detection techniques.

- Your martial arts instructor announces that tomorrow you're going to work on ways to defend yourself against multiple attackers.
- Your police defensive tactics instructor tells you that this afternoon you're going to work on prone handcuffing techniques.

Upon receiving the advanced notice, you imaged certain specific sights, sounds, physical sensations, smells, and even tastes as it relates to the training. You might have imaged these things for several minutes or for no more than a few seconds. In this book we expand on this natural process and enhance it to make you a better warrior.

Four examples of the power of mental rehearsal

Example 1:

This one has been around for years so you might have already heard of it, but it's worth repeating.

Australian psychologist Alan Richard conducted a small experiment on basketball players. After ensuring they all possessed equal free throwing skills, he divided them into three groups and organized them as follows:

- The first group would physically practice free throws every day.
- The second group would only visualize themselves doing free throws.
- The third group wouldn't do anything at all.

The result after a few weeks shocked Richardson and his crew. Upon testing them, the group that physically practiced and the group that practiced visualization were nearly comparable. The group that did nothing during the study didn't improve at all.

I believe if the visualization group had used *mental rehearsal* techniques, which bring into play all of the senses, they would have scored even closer to the group that practiced physically.

Example 2:

Dr. Lawrence Miller is a clinical and forensics psychologist and law enforcement trainer. In an article that appeared in *Police One* titled, "Mental Toughness for Law Enforcement," he wrote this about mental imagery.

"The ability to mentally project oneself into a different mindset or situation is a time-honored psychological technique for enhancing skill in sports and the performing arts, and only quite recently has this begun to be specifically applied to law enforcement training. Multisensory mental rehearsal exercises can be used to:

- simulate training scenarios.
- enhance real-world skills.
- analyze and correct errors.
- mentally prepare for action.
- enhance overall confidence.

"Mental rehearsal can be combined with real-life training to enhance performance in the field."

Example 3:

During the war in Vietnam, a South Vietnamese Army soldier and an accomplished artist, was captured by the North Vietnamese and incarcerated in a horrific military prison. Because he didn't have paint supplies, he would mentally "paint" throughout the days and nights of brutality and starvation. Later, and while still in captivity, he was able to acquire burnt chunks of wood and would sketch on whatever he could find. To his happy surprise, he had retained his skill, though his captors had broken his hand and never repaired it. Today his art is featured in art shows throughout the Northwest.

In another example, an American prisoner of war, a passionate golfer, would mentally practice his shots during his years of captivity. Upon his release, he found he had lost only a little of his skill.

In the 25 years since I first found mental rehearsal, it has swept through the world of martial arts, law enforcement, and the military. Not everyone is doing it, of course, but more and more warriors have found the incredible power of this unique training tool. I firmly believe word will continue to spread by those who regularly practice it, including enlightened trainers.

Lots of ideas, technology, and training approaches come and go in the warrior community, with more things discarded than kept. What remains are those things that work.

Mental rehearsal works.

CHAPTER 1

MYTHS ABOUT MENTAL REHEARSAL

Myth 1: It's difficult

Do you remember what you did right after stumbling out of bed this morning? How about what you were doing just moments before reading this book?

For each of these questions you formed a brief or lengthy mental image of your activity. It wasn't hard because you've got lots of experience doing it. After all, you form mental images of things all day long: your spouses face, your dog's happy wiggle when it sees you, the sergeant's scowl, the shelf where the reports are kept, and your sensei's flawless sidekick.

You already know how to form mental images. Now you can tweak your innate ability a little to make you a better warrior.

Myth 2: It takes a long time to benefit

No it doesn't. From your very first mental rehearsal session you begin implanting your desired goal, whether it's a fast and smooth magazine change, an accurate punch combination, or a swift application of a police control hold.

After your second mental rehearsal session, you're a little smoother than you were after the first time you tried it.

Just imagine how much you're going to improve after half a dozen short sessions.

Myth 3: You have to sit cross-legged with your palms together

No you don't, but you can if you want. Mental rehearsal practice can be done anywhere and in almost any manner. I've done it sitting cross-legged in a formal place of meditation and behind the wheel of a police patrol car. I've done it backstage waiting to give a presentation and while pacing back and forth minutes before I was to compete in a martial arts tournament.

Olympic skiers do it at the top of a slalom course, power lifters do it before they hoist hundreds of pounds over their fragile skull, police and military snipers do it before taking a life-saving shot, cops do it before they execute a high-risk mission, and military leaders do it before they lead men into harm's way.

Some of these folks might very well do it while sitting in lotus position, but I'm betting the majority do it every other place but.

Myth 4: You have to get into a trance

Nope. This common myth is probably confused with meditation. Thing is, you don't have to get into a trance to meditate, either.

As you will learn in this book, you can practice mental rehearsal with and without meditating. Just know that there is nothing mystical, woo-woo, or trance-like about the process.

Meditation is simply a moment of mental quiet.
Don't let others tell you it's complicated.

Myth 5: You need to practice in a special place

When many people envision meditators, they think of robed monks in a candle lit monastery or hippies sitting at the feet of an East Indian guru. There is that, but there are other places unique to the needs of the warrior community.

- Sitting in your police cruiser.
- Sitting in your car before going into your training facility.
- Riding in the back of a truck.
- Manning a post.
- Sitting along the sidelines waiting to compete.
- Sitting at home in your easy chair or lying in bed.
- Waiting at the range to shoot.

Myth 6: It's too mysterious

Many people aren't convinced that mental rehearsal isn't a lot of hocus-pocus. Take it from a meat and potatoes guy who has no interest in abracadabra and presto! —it isn't any of these things. Many research studies—past, present, formal, and informal—have shown mental imagery to be effective in many areas of physical performance, from sports to the battlefield. You still have to practice physically—it's not a substitute for training—but when used in conjunction with physical practice it's been found to improve performance more than physical practice by itself. Mental rehearsal to your physical practice is like a vitamin enriched, heavy-duty protein drink to your bench presses and squats.

CHAPTER 2

WHY WARRIORS NEED TO PRACTICE MENTAL REHEARSAL

On the battlefield, in all its incarnations, anything that doesn't work is quickly discarded and forgotten. In the police business, there are always new inventions guaranteed to improve officer safety and to make the high-stress job easier. In the past, guns that shoot nets over bad guys and guns that encase crooks in glue-like foam were announced with great fanfare but quickly disappeared when reality proved them ineffective. The same is true in the military and martial arts. New and exciting innovations might look good on paper or in controlled demonstrations, but if they don't do as promised in the harsh reality of actual battle, they go in the round file.

While new innovations for the dojo, the battlefield, and law enforcement come and go, the warrior's mind remains a constant. Yes, there are days when you're convinced you left your mind in your locker or workout bag, nonetheless it will serve you if you've properly primed it ahead of time.

Mental training wasn't emphasized when I began martial arts training in the mid 1960s, or when I served in the Army in the latter part of the decade, or when I joined the police department in the early 1970s. Nor was there much in the way of knowledge on the subject. Happily, as the 1970s drew to a close, this was about to change.

As mentioned earlier, my first introduction to mental imagery was at a Chuck Norris seminar in the 1980s. He called it visualization. Up to that point, I'd never heard of it and therefore never considered it as a possibility. As described earlier, he used it to "prefight" a new competitor in his mind. How he said it has remained with me to this day.

> *Then when I got into the ring with my new opponent, I had the advantage because I had experience fighting him, but he didn't have experience fighting me.*

Here is how this applies to you:

- You have experience *mentally* fighting Billy Bob but Billy Bob doesn't have experience fighting you.
- You have experience *mentally* confronting a violent drunk in a bar, but he doesn't have experience confronting you.
- You have experience *mentally* kicking through the door of a hostile house in a battle zone, but the enemy on the other side doesn't have experience confronting you.

Such mental training gives you a "position of advantage," if you will. Here are a few other reasons mental rehearsal is such a powerful tool for the warrior community.

Mentally rehearse for competition and qualification examinations

Competition in this sense means competitive sparring or contact fighting for martial artists, shooting competition for law enforcement officers and soldiers, and any other form of competition in the warrior field. Mental rehearsal makes better competitors—period.

Correcting mistakes in technique

- Mental rehearsal can help you to stop dropping your hands when you kick and help you not lean too far forward when you punch.
- It can help you to stop jerking your trigger and gripping your weapon incorrectly.
- It can correct flaws in your ability to assess multiple injuries and to not be distracted during long hours of guard duty.

Rehearse strategies

Cops, soldiers, and martial artists rely on strategies—i.e., plans and tactics—to engage a threat with success. Mentally rehearsing strategies helps to keep them at the forefront of your mind, and to employ them at your very best.

Overcome mental glitches

A mental glitch is a nagging, reoccurring problem. For example:

- Maybe you always freeze on a particular move in your kata.
- When shooting, you always pull right.
- After disassembling your weapon, you have trouble reassembling it in the right order.

Maybe you've corrected these mental glitches in training but you revert back to them under pressure. Mental rehearsal helps you rid these glitches once and for all.

Increase self-confidence

Even the most skilled warrior has moments when he doubts his abilities. By mentally seeing, hearing, feeling, tasting, and smelling all aspects of your skill set, you're able to reinforce your abilities and erase any nagging doubts.

Improve motivation

Getting yourself out of the rack to train can sometimes be many times harder than the actual training. Never have you been more creative than when the sound of rain pattering against your bedroom window conjures a dozen reasons why you shouldn't put on your sweats and running shoes to go pound the bricks.

Mental rehearsal will help you stay motivated to do whatever is necessary to end the day better than you were yesterday.

Focus attention in training

To improve, you know you must remain focused no matter how many times you have executed a drill, performed a kata, shot a course, curled a barbell, and the myriad other things you do to stay sharp and to continue improving.

Mental rehearsal helps you stay on task by letting you "see" your goal.

Regulate anxiety

Do warriors have to deal with anxiety? Do one-legged ducks walk in a circle? Anxiety and fear are part of warrior life—but so is functioning with it. Mental rehearsal helps you to accept it, deal with it, and get the job done while the butterflies in your stomach are having a good ol' cowboy hoedown.

Cope with and recover from injuries

Wherever cops, martial artists, and soldiers gather for a coffee or beer, it doesn't take long before they begin comparing injuries and scars. Getting hurt is simply part of warriorhood and so is coping with it. Mental rehearsal helps you to keep going—to win the competition, to take down the felon, to survive the firefight—no matter how much you're hurting. Whine and whimper when the job is done.

CHAPTER 3

NUTS AND BOLTS ABOUT MEDITATION

Before we get into the meditation phase and mechanics of the many mental rehearsal techniques, here is some basic information that should answer any questions you have. I hope it convinces you just how easy it is and how it fits neatly into the warrior lifestyle.

Meditation Prepares Your Mind

Mental rehearsal works best when you first prepare your mind to be receptive through meditation. The caveat here are the words "works best." Mental imagery also works—albeit not as well—without meditating first. The good news is it's not a one or the other deal because you can incorporate both methods into your life.

You will learn several meditation and mental rehearsal methods applicable to warriors who don't want to go to a Zen monastery and sit on a cushion for hours at a time. If you discover, as many have, that you really enjoy meditating and mental rehearsal, you're going to learn ways to increase your time from a few minutes to 30.

You're encouraged to try all of the meditation techniques at least twice. You might stick with one method, and that's fine. Or you might choose two, three, or four ways to meditate so you have a choice depending on how you feel on a given day. Some "experts" agree with using more than one method and others don't. More on this later. What is important is you're able to induce a state of relaxation in which your mind becomes susceptible to positive input.

If A Method Works For You, It's A Keeper

If a particular technique works for your buddy don't assume it will work for you. It might and it might not. Your task is to find one for you.

It's All About Being Positive

Training your mind is all about keeping things productive, ever improving, and being at your absolute best. You already have negativity in your head, lots of it. Mental rehearsal is about erasing damaging, pessimistic, and unnecessary input, and replacing them with all that is positive and excellent.

Consider this a negativity-free zone.

When And Where To Do It

There are no set rules or requirements as to when and where to use mental rehearsal. If you already meditate, you can take advantage of your mellow mind and body and add rehearsal to the last few minutes of your session.

If you're in a situation where you're unable to meditate first, simply do one of the last three variations listed under the header above: "Variations of Mental Rehearsal." If you can't do mini movements where you are without drawing guffaws from your buddies, do one of the less obvious methods so no one knows what you're doing.

You can practice upon first awakening or before you go to sleep. You can do it sitting in a vehicle before a mission or over in the corner of a room before stepping into the ring. You might like doing it before breakfast or afterwards. You can do it in a bunker, tank, or while sitting in court waiting to testify.

It doesn't matter when and it doesn't matter where; just do it.

Here are the most common positions.

Sitting

If you've been meditating for a while, this is probably your first or second favorite position. Indeed, when most people think of meditation, they image a shave-headed monk in a robe sitting on a cushion, legs wrapped into an extraordinary knot, eyes closed, back ramrod straight, and hands folded together with thumbs touching. I call this the classic posture, easily identifiable by the position of the legs and feet—legs crossed and feet on the opposite thigh.

Some people can do the classic right off but others must work for months to develop the flexibility. As a martial artist I have above average flexibility but I can't sit this way. Oh I could … once, but it would take the fire department's Jaws of Life to get me out of it. I sit with my legs folded like a kindergartener.

If you can sit in the classic posture, then do so. If you can't but for whatever reason you choose not to work toward it, or doing so would draw unwanted attention when you're around people, don't worry about it. It's not that big of a deal.

It's important to sit with your back and neck straight because it's been shown to facilitate proper breathing. Millions of meditators over the last 2500 years agree. You might find this fatiguing; I did. This means you've found a weakness in your body. Keep at it and within a few weeks your back and neck will strengthen.

Where you sit is up to you. In a Zen temple, a chapel room, the hood of your vehicle, in your car, on the wing of a plane, on a sandbag, on a hill in Afghanistan, in a stinky locker room, or sitting in a clump of trees on a stakeout. Where you sit isn't important. It's far more imperative that your meditation and mental rehearsal are productive so when you're up and moving again, you're a little better at something for having practiced in your head.

Standing

Formal standing meditation is an excellent way to meditate and image, and it can be quite comfortable once you get into the groove. Perhaps marksmanship, kata, and learning legal statutes were uncomfortable in the beginning for you. Now you do these things easily. It's the same with standing.

As you will learn, you don't always have to stand formally. More casual ways, such as waiting in line is the perfect opportunity to practice. Do it while waiting for a bus, waiting to be seated at a restaurant, standing post, waiting to be called out to compete, and any other place where you normally stand or have the option of standing.

Depending on the place and situation, you can use one of the meditation methods in this book to calm yourself and ready your mind, or you can simply take a few deep, quiet breaths, and begin. If you can close your eyes without drawing unwanted attention, do so. If you have to keep them open, simply focus on something—far off terrain, your steering wheel, or the back of the guy's head in front of you—and image the activity in which you want to improve.

Lying down

Whether you're lying face down, on your back, or curled into the fetal position, you can meditate and practice mental imagery. Just don't fall asleep. If you do drift off every time you try to meditate when lying down, it's not a good position for you. It is when you want to relax and calm down but don't do it when you want to practice imagery.

How Long Should You Do It?

There is no set time limit. You can practice for 1 minute or 25. When I practiced formally in a temple, our sessions lasted 25 minutes with a 5-minute break. It wasn't a smoke 'em if you got 'em period but rather 5 minutes of vigorous walking meditation.

At the 25-minute mark, a gong would sound. We would get up, place the back of one hand into the palm of the other, and then walk fairly quickly around the outside of the sitting area. When the 5 minutes were up, the gong would sound again, at which time we would resume sitting formally on our cushions for another 25 minutes. At weekend retreats, we followed this pattern from 5 a.m. to 8 p.m. Was it hard? Ooooh yeah. Was it effective? Yes, and it was clear that a week or two of this—the length of some retreats, which I never did—would be extraordinary.

One-minute sessions are at the opposite end of the spectrum. I do these all the time during my writing day. I swivel my desk chair around, focus on a tree branch outside my window, and mentally image myself executing a combination, say a sidekick followed by a backfist. In reality the combo takes about a second and a half. So I image it at the same speed, getting in 20 repetitions or so. When I finish, I turn back to my computer, perspiration free, but with an ever so slightly better combo. At the least, I've kept the technique in the forefront of my mind.

Between 1-minute and 30-minute meditations are 5- 10- and 15-minute sessions. These fit well in the warrior's lifestyle.

Usually, how long you meditate and practice mental rehearsal depends on your circumstances. For example, if you're doing a session in your squad car before you kick in a door, you probably won't do it for 25 minutes. If you're sitting on a cushion before a flickering candle, you're likely to go longer than a 1 minute.

Whatever the time period, just do it. Do it once a day or do it 10 times a day.

Breathing

One writer said, "The breath is the current that connects body and mind." For our purposes, this means through slow, mindful breathing, you enable your mind and body to be receptive to your mental rehearsal. The breath calms the body and mind, and allows your images—proper shooting technique, courage to face a tough opponent, or staying alert on guard duty—to penetrate deeply into your mind.

Mindful breathing helps you to control your thoughts and to quiet your agitated mind so you're better able to learn, focus, observe, understand, visualize, image, create, and a host of other things applicable to today's warrior.

You got to breathe all day long, so why not improve how you do it to get the most out of it?

How Not To Breathe

Many people breathe incorrectly; some experts say most people do. The incorrect way is to inhale into your chest as opposed to into your belly. Chest breathing gets you through life but not without problems, such as irritable bowels, dizziness, apprehension, and unclear thinking, to name a few.

Who needs these things? Not you and not your buddy. So get him to read this too.

How To Breathe

If you've been a chest breather all your life, breathing into your belly takes a little conscious effort. It's worth it, though, because you benefit by getting things most chest breathers don't: more energy, better concentration, better digestion, and reduced stress and anxiety.

Beth Shaw, founder and author of YogaFit, said this:

Because most people have stressful work and lives, commonly they only use the upper third of their lungs to breathe. This "chest breathing" tends to be very shallow. Deeper, fuller "stomach breathing" is more beneficial for the entire body: It opens the blood vessels that are found deeper in the lungs to allow more space for oxygen to enter into the blood, and improves concentration and mental capacity. Stomach breathing can be learned and practiced through various breathing exercises.

Here is how to do it

Do this lying down, sitting, standing, skydiving, and shooting. In short, do it anywhere you normally breathe.

- Put your palm on your belly.
- Breathe as you do normally.
- If your hand doesn't move, you're breathing into your chest. Don't do that.
- If your hand does move when you inhale, you're doing it the right way.
- Breathe in slowly and deeply, and feel your belly rise.
- Exhale slowly and feel your belly sink.
- Repeat for as long as you want. Like, forever.

Use belly breathing with all the meditation and mental rehearsal exercises in this book. You won't forget because I'll remind you along the way.

Create A Trigger Word

You're on the road and you're hungry. You can swing into McDonald's and grab a burger in three minutes or you can drive all the way home and take another 15 minutes to cook dinner. Both satisfy your hunger but fast food gets you there a little quicker (but clogs your arteries).

Think of a trigger word as fast food but without the negative connotation. Okay, not the best analogy but bear with me.

A trigger word gives you a slight jumpstart to activate your subconscious into relaxing your body and calming your mind. The word can be anything you want. I use my middle name, Wayne, because I don't know anyone with that name and I seldom hear it. I also use the word "melt" because to my mind I often feel like I'm melting when my body and mind sink into that wonderful place of profound calmness.

To be clear, if you're banging heads with people at a heavy metal concert, your whispered trigger word isn't going to do anything for you. But when you settle into a seated position or settle yourself into a standing position in a fairly quiet place, thinking or whispering your word will envelope you in a cloak of tranquil relaxation.

How deep does your trigger word take you into calmness and relaxation? If I had to guess at a number I would say about 20 percent, sometimes more sometimes less.

Use your trigger word(s):

- to quickly bring on the meditative state.
- when you want to quickly get calm and collected in the middle of training or your job.
- when you're briefly distracted from meditating and you want to resume.

Keep in mind, these only work after you have implanted the trigger word into your subconscious, which you will do in a momant. For now, lets assume your word has been implanted. Here is a little more about the three ways you can use it.

To quickly bring on the meditative state

This works whether you're practicing sitting, standing, or lying meditation. It doesn't matter if you're sitting in a Zen monastery or sitting on a pile of rocks in Afghanistan. You simply assume whatever position you want and take one or two slow inhalations and exhalations to settle and collect yourself. Inhale once more. Then on the slow exhalation, think or whisper to yourself your trigger word. Do it again if you like.

Instantly your body begins to relax and your mind mellows. You can remain at this relatively shallow level to do your mental rehearsal or you can follow whatever meditation method you're using to sink more deeply.

This will be explained in greater detail later.

To bring on a mild sense of calm

I did a lot of public speaking at one time and I was never comfortable with it, that is, until I discovered the idea behind the trigger word. I would whisper it or say it aloud just before I was to speak, finding that it immediately calmed and centered me.

When I had time, I would first say the trigger word followed by a short mental rehearsal session. I would see myself speaking slowly (I have a tendency to talk fast when I'm nervous), articulately, and looking as if I knew what I was talking about. It worked like a charm and I still do it today before an interview.

In the same fashion, use your trigger word just before you spar a formidable opponent, before you make a traffic stop, or before you go on patrol.

To resume your meditation

You've used your favorite meditation method to get yourself profoundly calm and still. You're feeling wonderfully mellow *aaaand*—your cell rings in your pocket. Next session try to remember to shut it off but for now you want to recover from the jarring interruption and get back to that wonderful place where you were before Beethoven's 5th sounded on your phone.

Time for your trigger word.

First, do one or two breath exchanges to resettle yourself. Then think or whisper your trigger word. Pause for a few seconds and think or whisper it again. Do it once more, if you like. Your trigger word won't take you all the way to the same happy place—you will have to repeat your meditation technique to do that—but it will help you get there a little sooner.

Those are three main purposes of your trigger word. But remember, this only works after you have implanted your trigger word into your subconscious. Here is how.

Establishing your trigger word

Your trigger word must first be inputted into your subconscious using one of the meditation methods in this book or in *Meditation For Warriors*. Use any method you want as long as it relaxes your body and calms your mind, a state in which you are more receptive to suggestion. It's a simple one too. This is what I used:

"Whenever I whisper or think Wayne [my middle name], I feel a deep sense of calm and relaxation."

That's it. Pretty simple. Here is the procedure:

- Sit, stand, or lay down.
- After wiggling yourself comfortable, follow whatever meditation method you want to get yourself as mellow as you're able.

- Enjoy the feeling for a while, 5 minutes, 10, or longer.
- Then give yourself the suggestion. Whisper or think, "Whenever I whisper or think [insert your word], I will feel a deep sense of calm and relaxation."
- Pause for a few seconds to let the suggestion sink in. Then think or whisper it again. Repeat the process 4 or 5 times. If you want to do it 10 times, that is fine.
- The next time you meditate, repeat the suggestion.
- Even on those days when you don't feel you've achieved a deep state of meditation, give yourself your trigger word suggestion. It still works a little.

After repeating this process for about a week, give your trigger word a test run. You can do the test anywhere in your daily life but I suggest you try it first when you're meditating.

Get into your position, take a deep breath, let it out slowly, and think or whisper your word. If you feel a comfortable sense of relaxation, it worked. If you don't, test it again.

Sometimes the trigger word is inputted after just a couple of sessions, but other times it requires more. If it didn't happen the first time, don't sweat it. It might take a few sessions, but soon your trigger word will be charged and good to go.

What does it feel like when you say or think your trigger word and it works? What I feel and what others have said they feel is a sense of enveloping calm. This tranquil feeling sort of cascades slowly from the top of my head all the way to my feet, bathing me, if you will, in a most pleasurable sense of relaxation.

Imagine settling onto a lounge chair on a quiet beach, a warm sun and gentle breeze caressing your body. It's like that, minus the sand fleas.

Here are three issues most meditators experience. While they might seem to be annoying, you learn to accept them. Once accepted, they are no longer a big deal.

Things That Itch

The ol' itch is an interesting phenomenon. You get nice and settled, you're following your breath, and you're about to experience a wonderful session.

Then your nose itches. The side of your neck tickles. The growing bald spot on top of your head feels like there is a spider on it. Oh, there is another spot smack in the center of your back.

Do you scratch the spot? Ignore it? Can you even ignore an itch?

It depends. If you're meditating in a Zendo or a Buddhist temple, most say to ignore it. Others say if it itches, scratch it. One expert claims that we itch all the time but we're so busy we don't notice. But in meditation, a quiet, introspective time devoted to one's self, the itching becomes apparent and often magnifies.

The reality with these annoying itches is that most don't really, well, itch. It's in the meditator's head. Here is what usually happens. You feel the itch in your armpit or in the center of your chest. But when you go to scratch it, there is no satisfaction because the spot didn't really itch. Your mind created it and your mind convinced you it was real.

When I was sitting in a formal Zendo, I would try everything to will a phantom itch away because I wanted to prove to myself how disciplined I was. But on those rare occasions when I "knew" this time the itch was not psychosomatic, but real and getting increasingly more intense, I'd give in and frantically scratch the offending spot. Fooled again. Nine times out of ten there was no satisfaction because the itch had only been in my head.

So what to do?

Scratch it. If you find that the itch was just in your head, next time focus a little harder on your meditation and see if it doesn't go away on its own. It probably will.

I got all itchy just writing this section.

Things That Hurt

When I began meditation and sat on a cushion, I was convinced my spine was going to snap and my kneecaps were going to pop off and roll across the floor. Of the two, my back hurt the most. I'd sweat profusely and my torso would quiver as if I were a Chihuahua. I've weight trained since I was a teenager and I've practiced martial arts since 1965 so pain wasn't new to me. But sitting motionless for 25 minutes was agonizing. I stuck with it, though, because I knew the pain was a result of weakness in my back, an area apparently missed by all my exercises. It took about a month of sitting five to six days a week before it finally went away. "Pain is weakness leaving your body," goes the old saying.

My approach was to treat my back as I did any exercise and work it (meaning, sit up straight like a West Point Cadet) until my muscles grew stronger. In the end, I toughened my discipline and strengthened my spine. A two-for-one deal.

If you don't want to tolerate the pain, simply change positions. I didn't have this option sitting in a Zendo because any movement is a no-no. I still think this way when I meditate alone. But you don't have to. If it hurts to sit on the fender of your Humvee, scoot off and lean against it. If your legs cramp while meditating in a police car during a stakeout, scoot around until you're comfortable again. But once you've found a comfortable position, don't move again until you've finished meditating.

Ammo To Ponder

Before we progress to the meditation techniques, please consider the following suggestions. They aren't carved in stone—they almost are—but rather based on findings from experienced meditators, including your humble author.

As a warrior, many times you will practice meditation and mental imagery in settings that people outside our community would never consider. So as you read the following suggestions, which were written for regular, cushion-sitting meditators, keep in mind that you might have to modify them depending on your circumstances.

I'll make suggestions here and there to nudge you in this direction.

Be consistent

Meditate as consistently as your time and schedule allows. If you can, set aside the same time every day, whether it's 5, 10, or 30 minutes. If sometimes your schedule forces you to practice meditating and mental imagery erratically—once this week, three times next week—you still benefit, but your progress will come more quickly when you follow a regular schedule.

It's all about your breath

The first meditation technique in the next chapter is one in which you follow your breath. This is the foundation method in virtually all meditation programs because it quickly relaxes the muscles, slows your heart rate, and helps your focus your mind. I encourage you to work to make it your foundation method.

Warm up

When you know you're about to meditate for, say, 15 minutes or longer, circle your arms a few times, circle your hips 10 times to the left and 10 times to the right, and stretch your legs a little. This does two things: It prepares your body to sit motionless for several minutes and it tells your mind what you're about to do.

Know you might experience frustration

It's common to have moments of frustration. You might think, "Doing nothing and following my breath is crazy." Or, "I can't get my brain to slow down!" This happens to new and veteran practitioners alike. When it does, remember two things: One, frustration is common and is one of the things you want to control through meditation. Two, meditation works. This makes it worth the effort.

Try out different methods

You might love sitting meditation but occasionally try something new: standing, lying, eyes closed, eyes open, and so on.

Try to meditate in the same place

If you meditate at home, establish one room for it. It might be an entire room or one corner. If you're deployed, find a place where you can do it consistently: a bunker, backseat of a vehicle, empty airplane, or any place you frequent regularly. For the martial arts, try to do it in one corner of your training facility, at home, or in your car before you go in to train. For police work, do it at home, in your squad when all is quiet, or in the locker room before roll call.

Note: *Meditation is still effective when you don't have a regular place.*

Read a little about meditation

There are far too many books on the market that are full of woo-woo—becoming one with the universe, rubbing crystals, eating tofu and beansprouts—so you have to inspect a few to find one that speaks to you. It's worth the effort because knowledge is ammo.

Listen to guided meditation

You might find that occasionally following guided meditation is a nice change of pace. Check out YouTube.com to find one that works for you, voice-wise and length-wise. Once you've achieved a deep state, slowly and subtly (so you maintain your deep relaxation) turn off the sound source, and proceed with mental rehearsal practice.

Do one-minute meditations during the day

You don't have to do anything formal for these. Just pause for a moment, follow your breath, and enjoy the mellowness wash over you. I'll explain in greater detail later.

Use a candle or a weapon

Meditators often use a lit candle to focus their attention. You can do that or use an object of significance to you. Some focus on their weapon, their shoulder patch, whatever. It's a simple device to help you stay in the moment. More on this later.

Don't worry about it

If meditation is new to you, you might find yourself worrying about whether you're doing it right, about your wandering mind, your sore back, or about some of the bizarre thoughts and images that arise. These are common issues for everyone. In time, your mind might still wander and weird thoughts and images might still come up, but you won't worry about them because you know they will pass.

Be alert to a loss of interest

This happens to veteran meditators and especially to newbies. Should you start feeling this way, do whatever it takes to stick with your meditation. Recharge yourself by re-reading this book; listening to guided meditation; altering or completely changing your method; or re-evaluating the reasons you began meditating.

Meditation is a powerful tool for the warrior but it's not always an easy path—and that is okay. You trained hard for your martial arts belt. You worked hard to get accepted by the police department and survive the academy. You made it though the military's basic training and your advanced training.

Meditation is pretty easy compared to those things.

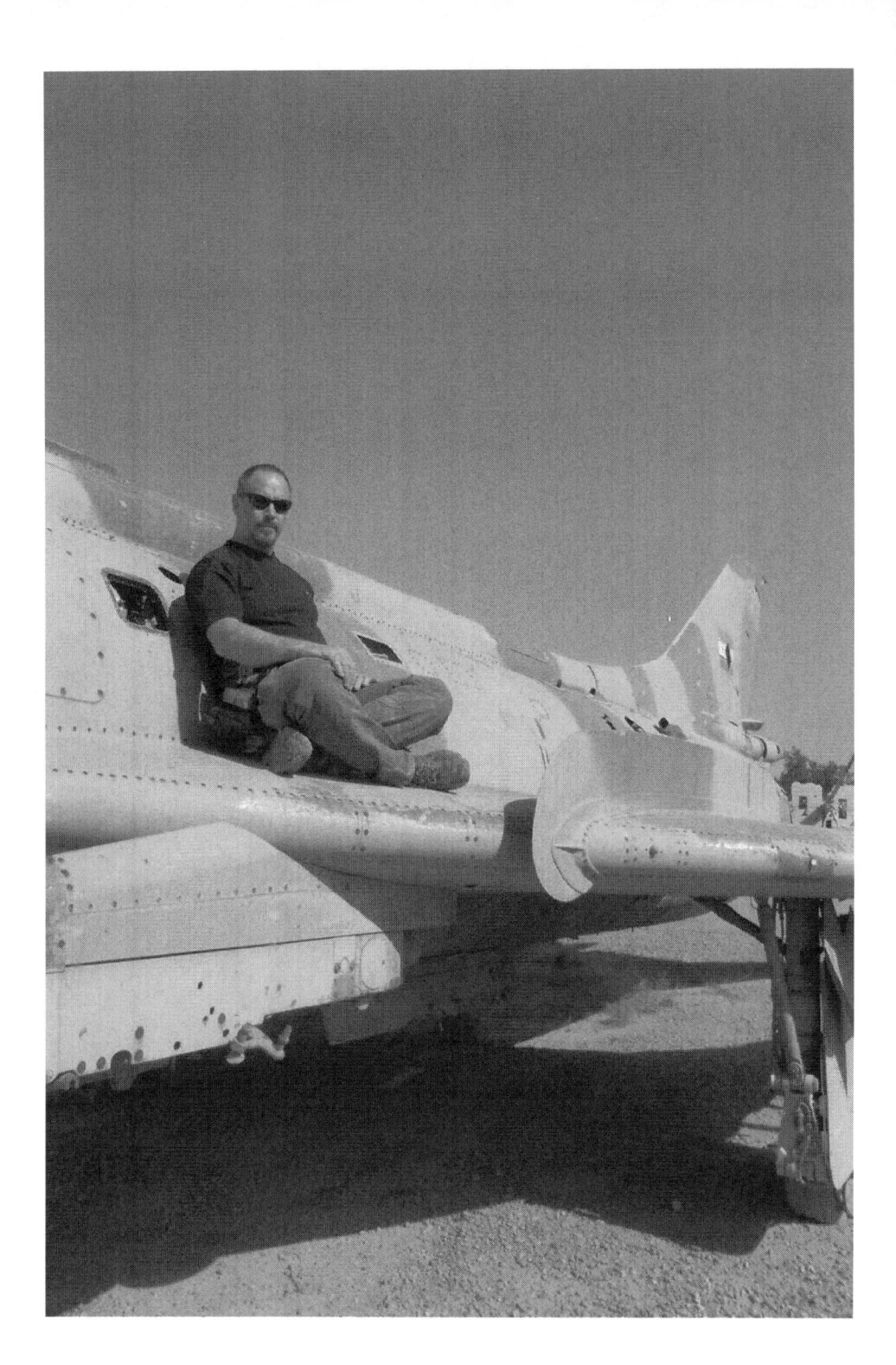

SECTION 2

Chapter 4: Introduction to Meditation Methods
Chapter 5: Meditation Techniques
Chapter 6: 60-Second Meditations

CHAPTER 4

INTRODUCTION TO MEDITATION METHODS

Do You Have to Meditate First?

Although this book is about mental rehearsal, you're getting a few meditation techniques too. This is because most if not all experts agree mental imagery practice is most effective by first calming your mind through meditation. The key words here are "most effective." This means mental imagery can be done without meditation, but the results won't be on the same level.

This isn't a problem. Sometimes in the warrior lifestyle you don't have time to sit and follow your breath. But there are still ways to do mental rehearsal to dramatically improve your objective. We will discuss this more as we proceed.

One Meditation Method Doesn't Fit All

You're getting several techniques in this section. Keep in mind meditation techniques are personal. Because Bill's way works great for him doesn't mean it will work for you. It might, but if it doesn't, as the saying goes, it don't mean nothin'.

So what do you do? Find one that does work for you.

No Such Thing as a Bad Meditation

In the Zendo, I was taught to never do more than one meditation method per sit. This is based in part on the belief there is no such thing as a bad meditation session. "Don't judge your sit," I heard often. It's all good; it all adds up; it's like a snowball rolling down a hill accumulating and accumulating. Staying with one method also helps to develop an ironclad discipline.

Sometimes all it takes is an adjustment to "fix" a session. For example, the problem might not be the actual meditation technique, but your initial setup. Say you're having trouble bringing on the first stage of calming the mind. The solution might be as simple as taking one or two extra calming breaths to start the process. Or perhaps you need to do progressive muscle relaxation (explained later) to "set the stage" before you proceed.

If I plan on sitting for longer than 10 minutes, I begin with a few neck, arm, and hip rotations. This stirs the blood a little and helps the muscles relax.

It's About What Works for You

The purpose of meditation for our purposes is to calm the mind and body so it's receptive to the mental imagery that follows. For this purpose, you can use any meditation method you like. It might be one that you're already using, one you found in *Meditation For Warriors*, or one of the methods in the following chapter. It doesn't matter as long as it relaxes your mind and body, and leaves you open to suggestion.

When You Want to Quit

There might be times when you don't want to meditate or when you want to stop early for any number of reasons: your back is cramping, your knee hurts, it's boring, it's too hot, too cold, or a killer bear is rampaging nearby. The human mind can be creative when coming up with reasons not to do something, especially if that thing is tough.

Just as there is no single meditation method that works for everyone, there is no single way to build an ironclad discipline.

Here are a few "devices" I've used and others have used to not quit:

- I tell myself: "People have been meditating for three thousand years. I can do it too."

- Mark off on a calendar every day you meditate. Those unmarked days scream volumes about your weakness.
- When you feel like ending a session early, give yourself three more minutes. When those are up, give yourself three more. When those are up and you still want to stop, then stop.
- If you've been routinely meditating for 15 or 20 minutes and you just can't face another session, do a 5-minute session. You will probably end up going longer but if you don't, at least you did it for 5.
- If you feel you can't focus on the meditation, then go ahead and begin the mental rehearsal. You still benefit from the practice, just not as much as when meditating first. Try not to do this very often.
- There will be times when you don't feel like meditating. This might be the result of a bad day, a headache, there is something good on TV, or you're starting to think it's a waste of time. Understand that these poor excuses are something every meditator must battle and, in fact, are the very reasons you *should* meditate.

"The benefits don't come from being good at it," says John Schaldach, curriculum and training coordinator at Mind Fitness Training Institute in Alexandria, Va. "They don't come from perfecting it. *They come from just doing it.*"

Remind yourself you're a warrior and as such you're above yielding to such sorry excuses. Warriors do what others can't. Warriors do what needs to be done. Warriors move toward what others flee from.

Meditate on those qualities.

How to End a Session

Whether you're just meditating for its pleasurable benefits or meditating to prepare your mind to be receptive to your mental rehearsal, it's always a good idea to come out of it slowly. You can do this a couple of ways.

- At the end of your session and before you open your eyes, tell yourself something similar to this: "I will now proceed with my day and carry with me this profound sense of calm and relaxation." If you have also practiced mental rehearsal, tell yourself something like this: "I will now carry into my day this profound sense of calm and relaxation, and the mental rehearsal skills I have just practiced." Phrase this so it applies to your situation.

- When you have an especially deep meditation session, tell yourself something like this: "I am going to slowly count backwards from 5 to 1, and on 1 I will awaken calm, relaxed, and better at [insert what you mentally rehearsed]." I did this last night. I went so deeply into my meditation I could barely move, nor did I want. I did the backwards count and on 1, I was alert and good to go.

CHAPTER 5

MEDITATION TECHNIQUES

In this chapter you will learn a few popular meditation techniques that can be done sitting, lying, and standing. You can use them solely to instill a calm mind and relaxed body before competition, heading out on a mission, or to "come down" from a high-energy and high-tension event.

For our purposes here, meditation is to increase your suggestibility to mental images. The calmer you are, the deeper the positive imprint.

So you're getting a two-for-one deal here.

SITTING

You can practice sitting meditation wherever you want, such as:

- on a cushion in a Zendo or Buddhist temple.
- on a cushion or chair in your home where you have established a place for meditation.
- anyplace else in your home you desire.
- on the hood of a military vehicle.
- in a police car.
- in an airplane.
- on a sandbag.
- in a noisy theater, sports stadium, or park.
- at a martial arts tournament or seminar.

- on the beach.
- any other place that allows you to bend in the middle and sit on your butt.

How long?

If you're meditating for its own sake, do it for a few seconds up to 30 minutes. However, if you're meditating to induce relaxation and calmness prior to your mental rehearsal, you should allow for a minimum of 10 minutes: five minutes for the meditating phase and five minutes for the rehearsal. If you allot, say, 20 minutes for your session, you can meditate for 10 and practice mental rehearsal for 10. Or meditate for 15 minutes and practice mental rehearsal for 5. There are exceptions in which you can do both for less than 10 minutes, which will be discussed as we proceed.

In one study, 48 Marines were divided into two groups before they deployed for war. Thirty-one practiced mindfulness meditation—focusing on the present, such as their breath—while the rest were used as the control group, meaning they didn't meditate. The meditating Marines practiced for only 12 minutes a day. Only 12 minutes! After eight weeks, the meditating Marines scored higher on mood and working memory evaluations.

You can easily do 12 minutes.

Is there a specific way to sit?

Nope. Sit anyway you want. If you can sit in lotus with your legs and feet in a knot that would make a sailor proud, go ahead. If you can only sit with your legs crossed like a little kid, do that. You can also sit on the end of a dock with your bare toes in the water, on a barrel with your legs dangling, or on a stack of ammo boxes.

Most teachers of meditation believe a straight back/spine is more conducive for proper breathing and bringing on the meditative state. I agree, but I also know there are many times in the warrior community when this isn't possible because it will draw unwanted attention. With this in mind, you're encouraged to sit with good posture as often as you can. But those times when you're around a lot of people, find a position that allows you to meditate without drawing catcalls.

Sometimes your posture is simply a matter of convenience. For example, if I'm slumped in my easy chair with our two little dogs on my lap when the urge to meditate hits me, I just do it without disturbing them. I still benefit and do so without enraging Boot and Rocky, two five-pound killer dogs.

One more thing about posture

When your upper torso is nice and straight, it's actually easier to breathe because there is more room for your lungs to work. It's also easy to feel all the many muscles involved—from your head to your toes.

Once you have developed the muscles to keep your upper body straight and tall, you will find good posture to be more comfortable than slumping like a teenager. Many times when I'm sitting and feeling so tired I just want to slump, I do the exact opposite and straighten my back. Though it's counter intuitive, I find sitting tall far more relaxing.

SITTING MEDITATION TECHNIQUES

The following method is presented as the first technique in my first meditation book, *Meditation For Warriors* because it's the basis from which other methods derive. I'm presenting it here again as the first method for the same reason. I have rewritten it a little in hopes to make it fresh to those readers who bought the first book.

Sitting Meditation 1: Basic Follow Your Breath Meditation

This method is found in all schools of meditation and is considered a foundation from which others stem. It's simple and all it requires is one thing: your breath.

I use this whenever I'm waiting to fill up the car, sitting on the sofa looking out the window, sitting on the porch watching the trees move in the wind, and at night to calm my nerves after a busy day.

Wherever I do it, I take a couple of deep breaths to relax and to convey to my mind and body I'm about to meditate for a few minutes. I whisper or think my trigger word two or three times to jump start the process, and then breathe normally as I follow my breath's path. In short order, sometimes less than a minute, I begin to feel calm, collected, and relaxed. But I don't stop; I continue to go deeper and deeper.

As you begin to follow your breath, forget all the drama in your life and all those tasks you have to do. Easy? No. You will be distracted and your mind will go off in a hundred directions. Don't fight it when it happens because you don't want to give those intruding thoughts too much credit. Instead, acknowledge them and return to following your breath.

- Get comfortable wherever you're sitting. Scoot a little this way and that way and wiggle your butt to get your sit-down muscles where you want them.
- Think or whisper your trigger word three times.
- Slowly inhale and exhale two or three times to settle your body and alert your brain as to what you're about to do.
- Tell yourself you're going to follow your breath for a few minutes to bring on an enjoyable sense of calm to your mind and body.

The above steps take a minute or two to do.

- As you inhale slowly, deeply, and quietly through your nose, follow your breath's path through your nose, down through your chest, and into your lower belly.
- Now follow your air as it moves out of your belly, up through your chest, and gently out your mouth.

Note: One cycle inhalation and exhalation will take between 10 and 15 seconds, or whatever is your normal breathing pattern.

- Repeat for 5 or 10 minutes. If you're really enjoying it and you want to go for 15 or 20 minutes, great! Do it.
- When you're done, proceed into whatever mental rehearsal you have planned.
- If you're meditating just to mellow out, tell yourself before you conclude that you will carry this wonderful sense of calm and relaxation into the rest of your day.

Key points:

- Breathe so quietly no one knows you're doing it, even if they are next to you.
- With each exhalation of your initial two or three breaths, feel your body grow progressively relaxed. Will yourself to make it happen.
- Don't breathe too fast or too slow. Breathe at the same pace you normally do.
- Got a cold or hay fever? Inhale and exhale through your mouth.
- Feel your lower belly swell with each inhalation, not your chest. This is key.
- You might feel as if you're not getting enough air. Long-time meditators experience this from time to time too. Don't be alarmed. It's just a feeling because you're suddenly more conscious about breathing. Just stay on task and focus on inhaling and exhaling at the same pace and volume you normally do.

Note: To reiterate, consider the above method your foundation technique. Most of the following methods are variations of this one. Master it.

Sitting Meditation 2: 4-Part Breath
(not to be confused with 4-count breathing)

A nice side benefit with this method is how well it relieves stress and oxygenates your blood. The combined effect helps to calm your mind and helps you feel better physically.

- Get comfortable wherever you're sitting. Scoot a little this way and that way and wiggle your butt to get your sit-down muscles where you want them.
- Think or whisper your trigger word three times.
- Take two or three deep breaths to settle your body and alert your brain as to what you're about to do.
- Tell yourself you're going to follow your breath for a few minutes to bring on an enjoyable sense of calm to your mind and body.

Now you're ready to begin the breathing pattern.

- Part 1) As you inhale once, feel the oxygen slowly expand your lower belly.
- Part 2) Then slowly expand your ribs.
- Part 3) Then slowly expand your chest.
- Part 4) Feel the air in your throat.

Without straining, hold the air in for 10 to 15 seconds. Now reverse the process.

- Part 1) Feel the air slowly leave your throat.
- Part 2) Then slowly leave your chest.
- Part 3) Then slowly leave your rib area.
- Part 4) Then finally slowly deflate your belly.
- Repeat this breathing pattern for as long as you like.
- When you're done, proceed into whatever mental rehearsal you have planned.
- If you're meditating just to mellow out, tell yourself before you conclude that you will carry this wonderful sense of calm and relaxation into the rest of your day.

Key Points

- Although there are 4 parts to your inhalation, you're breathing in only once.

- Since the inhalation and exhalation are done in stages—in: belly, rib area, chest and throat, then hold. Out: throat, chest, rib area, belly—it forces you to stay in the moment. That means you must focus on pace and where your breath is.
- Do not take in more breath or less breath than you normally do. Breathe quietly.
- Should you feel dizzy, you're probably breathing too rapidly or too deeply. Simply breathe normally but in the described stages.

Sitting Meditation 3: Candle Or Light Meditation

Having been a cop and a soldier, I advise you not to set up a candle in your PD locker room or on your tough box (that's the modern day Army footlocker for you old timers) because you will never hear the end of it. I suggest you save the candle for home meditation.

Instead, use a light. It can be a hanging light bulb, a distant light on a building, a blinking beacon, or any other one that is fixed and far enough away to not hurt your eyes.

Candle

Turn off the lights, but leave on a hall light or nightlight so your room is semi-dark. Position the candle as close to eye level as possible. It should be comfortable to look at it.

Light

The light should be easy for you to see. You don't want to have to crank your neck to see it or twist around in your seat.

Comfort is stressed here because the candle or light is a just a device to facilitate your meditation. You don't want to have to think about it; you just want to gaze at it.

- Get comfortable wherever you're sitting. Scoot a little this way and that way and wiggle your butt to get your sit-down muscles where you want them.
- Think or whisper your trigger word three times.
- Take two or three deep breaths to settle your body and alert your brain as to what you're about to do.

Now you're ready to start your meditation.

- Look at the candle or light.
- Breathe deeply into your belly and slowly exhale while looking at the candle or light.
- Continue the process for however long you plan to sit.
- When you're done, proceed into whatever mental rehearsal you have planned.
- If you're meditating just to mellow out, tell yourself before you conclude that you will carry this wonderful sense of calm and relaxation into the rest of your day.

Key points

- The trick is to see the candle or light without thinking about it. Consider it as nothing more than a point to return to when your mind wanders.
- Inhale and exhale at normal pace. Always breathe into your belly.

Sitting Meditation 4: Double Breath And Tense

This is an interesting meditation technique that some people love and others dislike. Those who love it say it brings on a deep sense of mental calm and physical relaxation. Those who don't care for it say it's too busy. Please try it a few times before you pass judgment.

- Get comfortable wherever you're sitting. Scoot a little this way and that way, and wiggle your butt to get your sit-down muscles where you want them.
- Think or whisper your trigger word three times.
- Take two or three deep breaths to settle your body and alert your brain as to what you're about to do.

You're now ready to commence.

- Sharply inhale through your nose, one short inhalation followed immediately by one long one.
- Now tense your entire body, from your face to your toes and everything in between. Do it hard enough that your muscles tremble.
- Hold your breath and the tension for 5 or 6 seconds.
- Sharply exhale out your mouth, one short exhalation, followed by one long one.
- When you're done, proceed into whatever mental rehearsal you have planned.
- If you're meditating just to mellow out, tell yourself before you conclude that you will carry this wonderful sense of calm and relaxation into the rest of your day.

Key Points

- Think of the exhalation as forcing your body's tension out.
- Don't tense so hard your face turns red and you lose consciousness. Stop at the first indication of total body tension.
- Don't hold the tension and your breath longer than 6 seconds.
- Use this method whenever you want to bring on a pleasant sensation of physical relaxation.

Sitting Meditation 5: 8-count breathing

In *Meditation For Warriors*, I discussed the 4-count breathing technique, which in military circles is often called tactical breathing. I'm not calling it tactical here for the simple reason the term is so overused—tactical pants, tactical run, tactical lunch—that it's becoming a tad silly. "4-count" serves our purpose, plus its meaning is clear.

The 8-count is similar to the 4-count except … it's twice as long. Okay, there is a little more to it than that.

I've only been doing it in the months since I penned *Meditation For Warriors* but what I've found and really enjoy is that all the stages are slower paced than 4-count. Sometimes with 4-count I feel a sense of being hurried. I don't get that with 8-count.

Some meditators say they become calm faster with 8-count. That said, how quickly you feel the effects of meditation is based on many things, such as where your head is when you start, how favorable your environment is when meditating, whether you're ill or hurting, and many other things.

Does this mean you should give up 4-count? Not at all. The 4-count method is a powerful technique that the warrior community—as well as people outside of it, including those in the medical field—have used for years. Additionally, as I noted in an earlier chapter, what works for one person might not work for another. Some might like the slower pace of 8-count, while others might find they take in too much air or they run out of air on the exhale.

In the end, it's what works for you, not for your barber and not for me.

- Get comfortable wherever you're sitting. Scoot a little this way and that way and wiggle your butt to get your sit-down muscles where you want them.
- Think or whisper your trigger word three times.
- Take two or three deep breaths to settle your body and alert your brain as to what you're about to do.

You're now ready to commence.

- Breathe in slowly to a count of 8: 1, 2, 3, 4, 5, 6, 7, 8.
- Hold it in for a count of 8: 1, 2, 3, 4, 5, 6, 7, 8.
- Exhale out your mouth for a count of 8: 1, 2, 3, 4, 5, 6, 7, 8.
- Hold it for a count of 8: 1, 2, 3, 4, 5, 6, 7, 8.

This is one cycle. Repeat for as many cycles as you like.

- When you're done, proceed into whatever mental rehearsal you have planned.
- If you're meditating just to mellow out, tell yourself before you conclude that you will carry this wonderful sense of calm and relaxation into the rest of your day.

Key Points

- There is a small learning curve as to how much air you inhale and at what pace you exhale. Take in too much too quickly or exhale too quickly, you might strain the last two or three seconds. Don't worry, you will adapt after a couple of cycles.
- If after two or three sessions you find the 8-count too difficult, modify it to 6 count. But progressively increase the time to 7 seconds in each phase, and then to 8. This might take two or three weeks in each progressive stage. Don't strain, just get to 8 when you can.

Sitting Meditation 6: Talk To Yourself

I can hear you now. "Dude, I'm decked out in—swat gear, police uniform, MMA shorts, military cammo—and you want me to talk to myself?" Well, yes, sorta.

This might at first seem to be a bit woo-woo but try it anyway.

The good news is that you talk to yourself in your mind or, if no one is around, whisper to yourself. The second bit of good news is that once you get into the groove, which might take a few minutes or a couple of sessions, you will find as others have, hearing your voice is an excellent way to keep you focused in the moment.

- Get comfortable wherever you're sitting. Scoot a little this way and that way and wiggle your butt to get your sit-down muscles where you want them.
- Think or whisper your trigger word three times.
- Take two or three deep breaths to settle your body and alert your brain as to what you're about to do.

You're now ready to commence.

- As you slowly breathe in, think or whisper, "I am ..."
- As you slowly exhale, think or whisper, "... calm."
- When thinking or whispering, "I am ..." be aware of your entire body. Imagine your inhalation filling all of you, from your head down to your feet (though you're breathing into your lower belly).
- As you exhale and think or whisper, "... calm," imagine the air leaving your body from your feet up to your head. As it exits out your mouth, feel a sense of calmness wash over you.

Key points

- This method might seem a little complicated at first, but it really isn't. You will own it after just a few breath exchanges.
- Every time you think or whisper, "... calm," let your body tension go. Physically maintain your good posture, but mentally sag into yourself.

Sitting Meditation 7: Get Heavy

This is similar to the "Melting Face Meditation" in *Meditation For Warriors*, except with that one you focused on melting your face one section at a time. With "Get Heavy" meditation, you mentally and progressively make your body heavy one section at a time.

You can do it two ways: Start with your head and work your way down or start with your legs and work your way up. It doesn't matter as long as it works for you. What is important, however, is once you make one section heavy, you maintain its heaviness as you move on to the next section. This requires 100 percent of your attention.

What if you lose your focus? Easy fix. Say you've progressed down to making your torso heavy but you lost your focus for a moment and you no longer feel heaviness in your shoulders. Simply go back up and recapture the heaviness there before continuing with your torso.

It's no big deal to lose your focus. Just go back and fix it. It's part of the process.

- Get comfortable wherever you're sitting. Scoot a little this way and that way, and wiggle your butt to get your sit-down muscles where you want them.
- Think or whisper your trigger word three times.
- Take two or three deep breaths to settle your body and alert your brain what you're about to do.

You're now ready to commence. Let's start with your head and work down.

- Be aware of all four sides of your head and all four sides of your neck as you slowly inhale. Mentally make all sides heavy. Don't move anything. Just make your head and neck so heavy they feel like they are pushing into your shoulders. If it helps, think or whisper "heavy" as you exhale. Feel the increased weight for 2 inhalations and 2 exhalations. Strive to make your head and neck heavier each time you breathe out.
- As you slowly inhale, be aware of your shoulders and arms.
- As you slowly exhale, mentally make them heavy and so weighted down you can't possibly lift them. Feel the increased weight for 2 inhalations and 2 exhalations. Strive to make them heavier each time you breathe out.

- As you slowly inhale, be aware of all sides of your torso: chest, back, and abdomen.
- As you slowly exhale, mentally make all four sides heavy. Don't move anything; just make them so heavy they feel as if they are pushing into your pelvis. Feel this increased weight for 2 inhalations and 2 exhalations. Strive to make it heavier each time you breathe out.
- As you slowly inhale, be aware of your all four sides of your pelvis.
- As you slowly exhale, mentally make your pelvis heavy without moving it. Make it so heavy that it seems to be pushing into your legs. Feel this increased weight for 2 inhalations and 2 exhalations. Strive to make it heavier each time you breathe out.

Before moving on to your legs, scan your head, arms, torso, and pelvis to see if they still feel heavy. If they don't, repeat the sequence to make them feel heavy again.

- As you slowly inhale, be aware of your legs and feet: front, sides and back.
- As you slowly exhale, mentally make your legs and feet heavy without moving them. Make them so heavy they feel as if they are sinking into the floor. Feel this increased weight for 2 inhalations and 2 exhalations. Strive to make them heavier each time you breathe out.
- Repeat the entire process from head to toe as many times as you want.
- When you're done, proceed into whatever mental rehearsal you have planned.
- If you're meditating just to mellow out, tell yourself before you conclude that you will carry this wonderful sense of calm and relaxation into the rest of your day.

Key Points

- If you don't feel the heaviness in your body sections, continue with the entire procedure. It might take two or three sessions before you do.
- Of course you're not really gaining weight with this procedure (someone always asks). The sensation of heaviness comes from

your body giving up all the tension you pack around everyday.
- You might find it helpful to think or whisper "heavy" on each exhalation.
- If you have progressed from head to feet and want to reverse the process by going back up your body, do so.
- Once you master this one, you will look forward to the profound relaxation you experience with it.

Sitting Meditation 8: Survey Your Body; Relax Your Body

This is similar to "Sitting Meditation 7: Get Heavy," but there are enough differences to warrant it being a separate method.

All of us—newbie meditator and veterans—experience periods when it's hard to control the monkey mind. You're on your third inhalation and exhalation sequence and there goes your mind—you're suddenly at the shooting range; you're having a black belt fantasy; or you're catching an *America's Most Wanted*. You bring your mind back to your breath but on your fifth exhalation, your brain is off to the mall. You bring your mind back to your breath but 20 seconds later your mind is off to …

However, with this meditation method, your mind is too busy checking out each body part to buzz off somewhere.

The survey process is simple. You're going to mentally section off your body from your head to your feet and evaluate each one until you have scanned your entire body. This method takes a little longer than the others so allow for at least 20 minutes, which includes your mental rehearsal.

Think of this as a two-part process.

Part 1: The first time you survey from your head to your feet, your objective is to only be aware of your various parts. If you feel any degree of discomfort, don't do anything other than be aware of the sensation.
Part 2: The second and, if you want, third time through, your objective is to use your mind to relax each body part.

Begin by thinking of your body as separated into the following sections.

Head and neck
Shoulders,
Arms
Hands (what they are touching)
Chest and back
Pelvis, front, sides
Rear (what it's touching)
Upper legs
Calves
Feet (what they are touching)
Let's begin.

- Wiggle your butt into whatever you're sitting on: sandbag, vehicle roof, car seat, workout bag, and so on. Straighten your spine and lengthen your neck. If you're naturally a slumper, please try sitting with a straight spine for this session. But if doing so might bring unwanted attention to yourself, sit as straight as you can without causing a scene.
- Inhale slowly, deeply, and quietly into your belly, and then slowly exhale. Do two or three cycles, allowing your breath exchanges to begin calming you.
- Whisper or think your trigger word. Repeat it two or three times and enjoy the feeling of relaxation wash over your body.

That is the prep. Now for the meditation.

- Be aware of your head and neck, front, sides, back, and top. See and feel them in your mind—every rise, fall, curve, and bump. If you have a twinge in a tooth, be aware of it. If you have a slight headache, be aware of it. If you're feeling good, be aware of it.
- Be aware of your shoulders, front, sides, and top. See and feel their shape. If tension is making you hold them high, ignore it for now.
- Be aware of your arms, upper and forearms. See and feel their shape. If you have a pain in one or both of them, just be aware of it.
- Be aware of your hands, back, top, and fingers. Be aware of what they are touching. If they are resting on your knees, feel the cloth of your pants. If they are folded into the classic meditation position—back of your left hand lying in the palm of your right hand, thumbs gently touching—feel the skin-to-skin contact.
- Be aware of your chest, back, and abdomen. See and feel their shape in your mind. If your stomach feels uncomfortably full or hungry, be aware of it. If your back hurts from sitting, just be aware of it.
- Be aware of your pelvis, front and sides. See and feel its shape.
- Be aware of your rear. See and feel its shape. Feel whatever you're sitting on—the rough hardness of a sandbag; the contours of an ammo box; or the hard discomfort of a wooden chair.
- Be aware of your upper legs. See and feel their shape and how they are positioned. Be aware of whatever the backs of your legs

are touching. Be aware of any pain in your legs.
- Be aware of your calves. See and feel their shape in your mind.
- Be aware of your feet. See and feel their shape. Feel whatever is on your feet. If you're barefoot, feel what they are resting upon.

This completes the survey and awareness stage. If you want to repeat this phase, please do.

For the second phase, you're going to repeat the same process, but this time you are to relax and soften each part. Do this with your mind and with your breath.

- Be aware of your head and neck, front, sides, back, and top as you inhale. Each time you exhale, see and feel your muscles, tendons, and skin melting over your skull into deep relaxation. Repeat two, three, or four times.
- Be aware of your shoulders, front, sides, and top as you inhale. As you exhale, feel your shoulders sink and grow heavy. If you normally carry tension and stress in them, repeat the inhalation and exhalation as many times as needed to completely relax the area.
- Be aware of your arms, upper arms and forearms as you breathe in. Each time you exhale, feel them become profoundly heavy and relaxed. Repeat two, three, or four times.
- Be aware of your hands, back, top, and fingers as you inhale. As you exhale, see and feel them become so light they could float upward. Repeat two, three, or four times.
- Be aware of your chest, back, and abdomen as you inhale. Each time you exhale, see and feel them sink and relax. If you're sitting with your spine straight, relax into it without allowing it to slump. Repeat two, three, or four times.
- Be aware of your pelvis, front and sides as you inhale. Each time you exhale, see and feel it grow heavier and heavier. Repeat two, three, or four times.
- Be aware of your butt as you inhale. Each time you exhale, feel it become heavy as it sinks into whatever it's sitting on. Repeat two, three, or four times.
- Be aware of your upper legs as you inhale. Each time you exhale, see and feel them become heavy and sink into whatever they are touching. Repeat two, three, or four times.

- Be aware of your calves as you inhale. Each time you inhale, see and feel them relax and become heavy. Repeat two, three, or four times.
- Be aware of your feet as you inhale. Each time you exhale, see and feel them grow heavy as they sink into whatever they are touching.
- Repeat the relaxation phase as often as you like.
- When you're done, proceed into whatever mental rehearsal you have planned.
- If you're meditating just to mellow out, tell yourself before you conclude that you will carry this wonderful sense of calm and relaxation into the rest of your day.

You might find as others have that your face continues to melt as you progress through your body. For example, you might be focused on relaxing your chest and back on each exhalation, and discover your face relaxing more too. This is fine. In fact, it's great. Don't fight it; enjoy it.

Key Points:

- Many find that body scanning is an easy way to appreciate mindfulness. Remember, mindfulness is the power of becoming fully aware of the present moment—non-judgmentally—rather than dwelling in the past or projecting into the future.
- If you carry extra tension in your shoulders, neck, and upper back, spend more time relaxing these parts.

STANDING MEDITATION

When doing standing meditation, you can use all the methods described above in "Sitting Meditation." However, if you're new to this, do only Sitting Meditation 1 and 2 when standing. Save Sitting Meditation 3 through 8 until you are more experienced.

The Classic Standing Posture

You can do standing meditation while assigned to a post, waiting in line, waiting for a bus, waiting for your spouse, and any other time you find yourself standing for a few minutes. Initially, it's best to practice what I call "The Classic Standing Position." Then once you understand the "rules" and feel comfortable with the process, you can do it more casually anywhere and anytime you're standing.

Here is the Classic:

- Find a quiet place to practice. Inside or outside, it doesn't matter as long as you won't be disturbed or distracted. Eventually, this won't be an issue.
- Stand with your feet about hip distance apart and your toes pointing forward. Don't lock your knees because it weakens your stance.
- Look forward with your head centered above your spine.
- Relax the muscles in your face, head, neck, and throat. Put the tip of your tongue just behind your upper teeth.
- Place your palms over your lower abdomen a couple inches below your navel. Your finger tips point toward each other, similar to how your hands would be if wrapped around a small post (or a huge post if you're a beer drinker). There should be a small space between your fingers.
- Inhale deeply into your belly and exhale completely. Repeat two or three times and make small adjustments in your stance, posture, spine alignment, and foot position to ensure your comfort and stability.
- Now just breathe normally.

Consider the Classic your basic foundation stance when standing. Now let's look at ways to meditate.

Standing Meditation 1: Follow Your Breath Meditation

If you're new to standing meditation, begin with the method described earlier in "Sitting Meditation 1: Basic follow your breath meditation." It's simple, easy to do, and since you have to breathe anyway, it's a good place to begin.

I use this breathing method when standing in public because no one knows I'm doing it. I also do it before going to bed after doing what I call my "perimeter check," in which I ensure the doors are locked and the yard is clear of crazed killers. I then stand in the dark and meditate for a few minutes. It's a nice way to shut off the day and prepare to sleep.

Here is how to do it:

- Stand straight and tall and place your palms on your lower belly, the fingertips of your right hand touching the fingertips of your left.
- Think or whisper your trigger word three times.
- Take a couple of deep breaths and feel a soothing sense of relaxation sweep through your face, shoulders, torso, and legs.
- Think or whisper, "calm" or "relax" on each exhalation.

You're now read to commence.

- As you inhale slowly, deeply, and quietly through your nose, follow your breath's path from the tip of your nose, down to your lower belly.
- Now follow your air as it moves out of your belly, up through your chest, and gently out your mouth.

Note: One inhalation and exhalation will take between 10 and 15 seconds, or whatever is your normal breathing pattern.

- Repeat for 5 or 10 minutes. If you're enjoying the process and your situation allows, go for 15 or 20 minutes.
- When you're done, proceed into whatever mental rehearsal you have planned.
- If you're meditating just to mellow out, tell yourself before you conclude that you will carry this wonderful sense of calm and relaxation into the rest of your day.

Key Points

- Think or whisper "calm" or "relax." Don't mindlessly think it or whisper it but rather ponder what the word means and image how it feels in your body.
- Stand as motionless as you're able. This might be hard but you will improve over time. If you absolutely have to move, make the adjustment as subtly as possible.

Standing Meditation 2: Progressive Relaxation Meditation

Some people require a few sessions to get into the groove of progressive relaxation, which is fine. It's worth the extra effort. Doing it while standing is similar to doing it while seated with one minor caveat. If you relax your body 100 percent, you will crumple into a pile. So think in terms of relaxing your body around 90 percent.

- Stand straight and tall and place your palms on your lower belly, the fingertips of your right hand touching the fingertips of your left.
- Think or whisper your trigger word three times.
- Take a couple of deep breaths and feel relaxation sweep through your face, shoulders, torso, and legs.
- Think or whisper, "calm" or "relax" on each exhalation.

You're now ready to commence.

- Here is an alternative to placing your palms on your lower belly. Instead, round your arms and hold your hands in front of your lower belly. Your hands are about 12 inches apart and between 12 and fifteen inches out from your belly. It's as if you're holding a beach ball in front of you.

Unnecessary tip: Don't do the beach ball position if you want to be unnoticed.

- If you get tired holding the invisible beach ball, but you want to continue meditating, place your palms on your belly as you did in the first standing meditation. With continual practice you will get stronger.
- Maintain a relaxed curve to your arms, whether your hands are resting on your belly or holding an imaginary beach ball.
- Keep your eyes open and fix your gaze on something in front of you.
- Maintain a straight neck, as if an attached string is pulling your head upward.
- Don't lock your knees.
- Breathe in slowly through your nose. Exhale slowly through your mouth and think or whisper "calm" or "relax" as you allow the

tension to leave your face and neck. Repeat two or three times.
- Breathe in slowly through your nose. Exhale slowly through your mouth and think or whisper "calm" or "relax" as you relax all the tension out of your shoulders. Repeat two or three times.
- Breathe in slowly through your nose. Exhale slowly through your mouth and think or whisper "calm" or "relax" as you relax all the tension out of your chest, back, and abdomen. Repeat two or three times.
- Breathe in slowly through your nose. Exhale slowly through your mouth and think or whisper "calm" or "relax" as you relax all the tension out of your pelvic area, front, sides and back. Repeat two or three times.
- Breathe in slowly through your nose. Exhale slowly through your mouth and think or whisper "calm" or "relax" as you relax all the tension out of your legs and feet. Repeat two or three times.
- Repeat the cycle as many times as you like.
- When you're done, proceed into whatever mental rehearsal you have planned.
- If you're meditating just to mellow out, tell yourself before you conclude that you will carry this wonderful sense of calm and relaxation into the rest of your day.

Key Points

- Mentally feel each body part relax as completely as possible.
- If the words "calm" and "relax" don't work for you, choose ones that do, such as "melt," "soften," or "heavy" to connote in your mind the release of tension. Hey, "release" is a good word too.

Note: We will look at a couple of casual standing methods when we look at ways to practice mental rehearsal.

CHAPTER 6

60-SECOND MEDITATIONS

Before we move into mental imagery techniques, let's look at three, one-minute meditations to help you achieve a mild sense of calm and relaxation when you're absolutely limited on time.

Use 60-second meditations as stand-alone:

- when you want to mellow out during a work break.
- when you want to "come down" after a chaotic incident.
- when you want to calm your mind and body before you engage in a potentially chaotic incident.

Use 60-second meditations to prepare your mind for a short mental rehearsal, such as when you are about to:

- give a presentation.
- go on a mission.
- engage in competition.
- be chewed out by a superior.

Here are three 60-second meditations:

60-Second Meditation 1: Flex Your Muscles

The technique can be done without drawing attention to yourself, unless you flex so hard you tremble like a lap dog.

- Sit or stand and get comfortable.
- If standing, allow your arms to hang free, or place them on your abdomen. If sitting, place your hands on your knees or thighs.
- Close your eyes or fix your gaze on a spot for one minute.
- Inhale slowly and deeply into your belly and slowly release it. Do this twice.
- Now inhale slowly and hold your breath as you tense every muscle you can from your feet to your face.
- Keep holding in your breath and keep tensing your muscles for 5 to 10 seconds. Don't allow any muscle to relax.
- Slowly exhale, and as you do, relax your muscles progressively in this order: face, neck, arms, shoulders, torso, hips, legs, and feet.
- Slowly inhale and exhale two more times without tensing your muscles.
- That is it. One time through.
- Tell yourself you will now carry your new sense of calm into your day.

Key Points

- Don't do the procedure too slowly or too quickly. When done as described, it takes 60 seconds, give or take 5.
- When exhaling, you must pay attention to what you're doing so you don't relax all your muscles at once. Strive to relax each body part in the order described.

60-Second Meditation 2: Push-And-Pull Breathing

This is one I've used in my martial arts classes for decades. I often conclude a class with several minutes of fast and furious drills in which I encourage students to bring out their inner rage. As the instructor, it's always fun to see even the mildest and meekest student turn into a pissed off mountain cougar as a result of whatever he or she is bringing to the surface and infusing into their techniques.

I don't want to turn them loose in that state of mind on our highways and byways so we do the following for 60 seconds, or for a couple of minutes if needed.

- Stand up straight with your feet about a foot apart.
- Lightly hold your hands palms up below your belly button about an inch away from your torso, fingertips slightly overlapping. It's as if you're holding the bottom of a bowl.
- Breathe in slowly as you simultaneously lift both hands up your body, as if lifting the bowl up to your chest.
- At chest height, roll your hands over and separate them. Your palms are now facing forward, your fingertips pointing upward in preparation to push outward.
- Exhale as you push your air outward, stopping just before your elbows lock.
- Roll your hands over until your fingertips touch and your palms face back toward you.
- Inhale as you draw your hands back to your chest, as if gathering fresh oxygen. Stop when they are an inch from your chest.
- Rotate your palms downward. They should be about four of five inches apart.
- Exhale as you lower your hands and push the air back to where you began.
- Rotate your hands until you're once again holding the bottom of the bowl.
- Repeat until the minute is up or go longer if you like.
- Tell yourself you will now carry your new sense of calm into your day.

Key Points

- The hand motions are nothing more than guides to keep you focused on your breathing. Imaging the motions as drawing in fresh air and pushing out old air can be helpful.
- Do the hand motions slowly. Go too quickly and you might get dizzy.

60-Second Meditation 3: Listen To Your Breathing

This 60-second technique requires that you listen to your breathing, noting how the air sounds different when passing into your nose from when it passes out of your mouth. Just notice, that's all you got to do. It's about focus and being mindful in the moment. When you aren't thinking or worrying about the past or the future, all that is left is right here, right now.

- Sit or stand and get comfortable.
- If standing, allow your arms to hang free, or place them on your abdomen. If sitting, place your hands on your knees or thighs.
- Inhale into your nose and listen to the sound.
- Exhale out your mouth and listen to the sound. If it sounds the same, that's fine. If it sounds different, that's fine too. Don't judge the sound; just hear it.
- Do this for 60 seconds.
- Tell yourself you will now carry your new sense of calm into your day.

Key Points

- Breathe normally. Go too fast and you might get dizzy.
- You can do 6 - 8 breath exchanges in a minute.

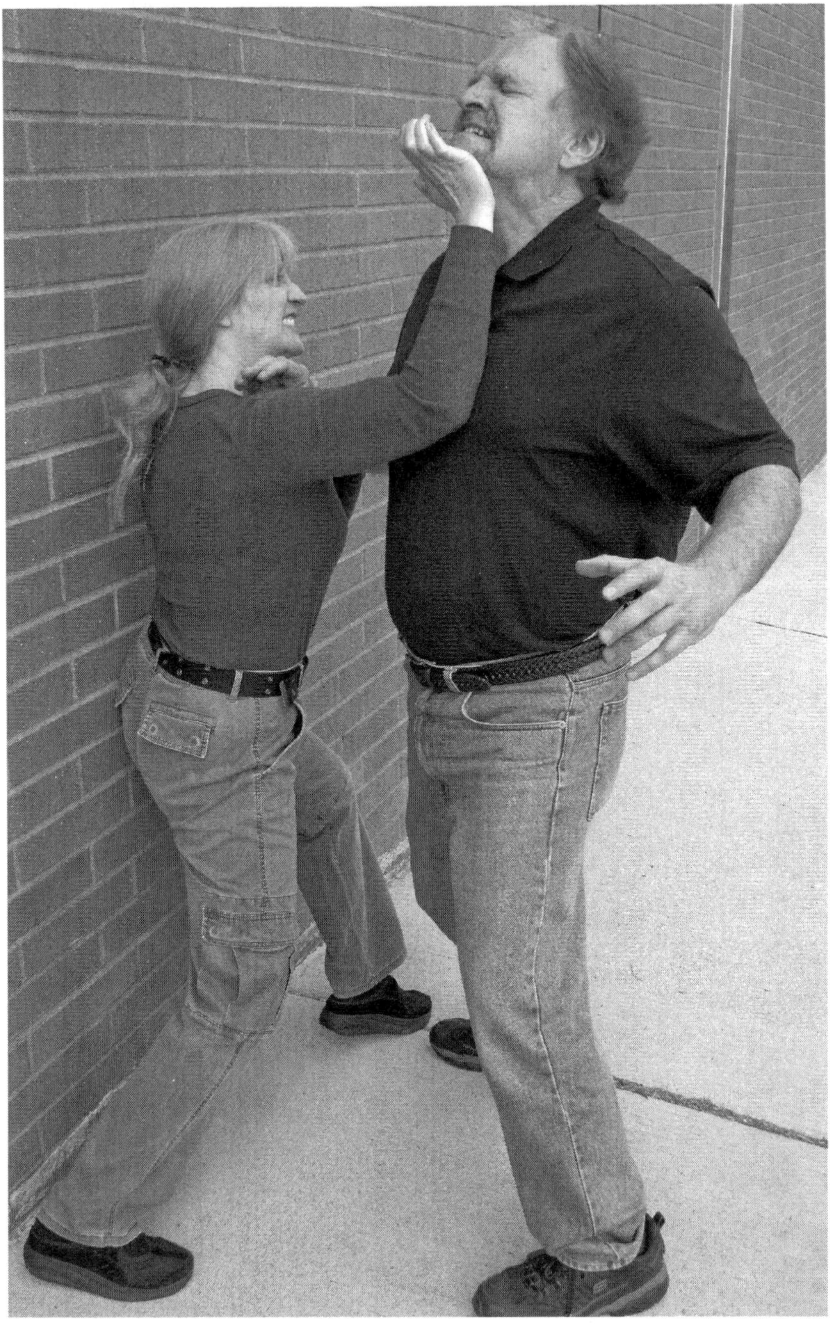

SECTION 3

Chapter 7: Introduction To Mental Rehearsal
Chapter 8: Nuts And Bolts of Mental Rehearsal
Chapter 9: Mental Rehearsal Methods
Chapter 10: Mental Rehearsal Without Meditation

Bonus: Chapter 11: Mental Rehearsal For School Teachers

CHAPTER 7

INTRODUCTION TO MENTAL REHEARSAL

How cool is this?

Around 1980, I attended a seminar by Frank Zane, who had won virtually every bodybuilding contest in existence, including the coveted Mr. Universe and Mr. Olympia. He was considered, and still is, a profoundly cerebral bodybuilder and hardcore proponent of the power of the mind. At the seminar, he talked about the necessity of using one's mind to image goals, such as "seeing" the muscle expand and contract and "feeling" it grow with each workout. I remember he had everyone on the edge of their seat when he talked about how some bodybuilders had developed fantastic abdominal muscles—ready for this?—without physically exercising.

I wanted to believe it but it sounded a little too far fetched.

But in 2007, a study appeared in an issue of *North American Journal of Psychology* about how athletes used mental imagery to practice hip-flexor exercises. At the end of the study, those who only imaged the exercises developed nearly the same strength gains as those who physically trained five days a week on exercise machines.

While this was a controlled study (I don't know if the one Zane was talking about was controlled), there are times when people are unintentionally surprised.

Here are two such examples. The first one happened to a friend and the second happened to me. Neither of us planned on the positive results or expected them. If we had, we would have done them more formally. Imagine the results then.

War story 1

Tom was a veteran bodybuilder and police officer who had developed fantastic strength and muscle size. For example, he performed flies with 85- to 90-pound dumbbells. This is where you lay on your back holding two dumbbells overhead and slowly lower them with slightly bent arms out from your sides, as if bear hugging a very large opponent.

After hurting his shoulder during a violent arrest, his physical therapist began training him as if he had never lifted a weight in his life. He was so debilitated and in such pain he had to do his flies without dumbbells. He went from 85 pounds in each hand to only the weight of his clenched fists. After a few weeks, though, he progressed to 1-pound dumbbells and, after three or four more weeks, he leaped all the way up to 2-pounders.

As he executed the painful, lightweight exercises, he would image the "toy" dumbbells to be the same monster weights he had used prior to his injury. He drew upon his memory of the gnarly feel of the steel handles biting into his palms, the way the weight strained his shoulders and arms, how his chest looked as it stretched on the down motion and flexed on the up, the smell in the gym, and the voices of other lifters in the room. In his mind and in his senses, he was lifting huge weights but in reality he was hoisting those little pink ones.

By the time he had progressed to almost 5-pounders, he discovered something that shocked him. The veteran lifter who had been reduced to exercising with a fraction of the poundage he was used to was actually making muscle size gains. Incredibly, his pectoral muscles had grown past where his development was prior to the injury. He had added new muscle using little pink dumbbells.

And mental imagery.

War Story 2

For 24 of the 25 years I was a police officer with Portland, Oregon PD, I taught defensive tactics, which included baton, takedowns, handcuffing, striking, and various control holds. I taught it to in-service officers, recruit academies, reserves, and an assortment of outside agencies.

Although I prepared a general outline for the police classes, I never practiced the material. At one point, I became curious as to how I could retain an above average skill level (I'm being humble. I was actually pretty good) since I didn't practice outside of the classes.

When I began to study mental rehearsal, I found my answer, later supported by other instructors who had experienced the same thing. I discovered in the course of conducting hundreds of training sessions, I was unknowingly practicing informal mental rehearsal. When I saw techniques done correctly, I got free practice. When I saw an error and I corrected the student, I was again getting free practice. In short, I was getting in thousands and thousands of mental rehearsal repetitions.

To reiterate, my bodybuilder friend and I were not deliberately practicing mental imagery, though that is exactly what we were doing, albeit informally and without the benefit of calming our minds first. Once my friend and I realized how much we were benefitting, we immediately began including meditation and mental rehearsal as part of our training.

CHAPTER 8

NUTS AND BOLDS OF MENTAL REHEARSAL

Scientists believe that we humanoids experience reality and imagined actions virtually the same way. Doctor Aymeric Guillot, a professor at the University Claude Bernard Lyon in France says whether we walk on a mountain trail or only rehearse it in our minds, we activate many of the same neural networks. These are paths of interconnected nerve cells that tie what your body does to the controlling brain impulses.

This means by imagining yourself clearing a jammed weapon or performing a difficult kata, you can improve. This has been proven repeatedly in controlled studies and has been shouted from the rooftops by some of the world's top athletes, martial artists and, more recently, elite law enforcement officers and military personnel.

You Already Do It To Some Extent

You wake up on your day off and make a written or mental list in your mind as to how you want the day to unfold. You're going to read for an hour, jog four miles, clean the garage, take a shower, and eat lunch. In the afternoon, you're going to check out a couple of games on the tube. In the evening, as a way to apologize to your spouse for not mowing the lawn, you take her to a nice eatery.

Monday is back and chest day at the gym. On the drive, you think about adding 10 pounds to your lat machine pull-downs and 15 to your bench. If you still have energy, you might add a fifth set of bench presses. At the gym, you follow your preplan and even get in that fifth set.

Formal practice as described in a moment builds on what you do naturally.

Mental Rehearsal In Real Time

If that four-count kick/punch combination takes two seconds to do in reality, you must mentally rehearse it taking two seconds. If your new shooting course takes two minutes to complete, you must rehearse it taking two minutes.

Mentally rehearsing in real time allows you to do lots of repetitions. Think how many times you can rehearse your fighting combination and shooting course in 10 minutes.

Point Of View

Some people mentally rehearse an action as if seeing it from their eyes, which is called first person viewing. Others see themselves perform as if watching a character on a movie screen, called third person viewing. One study reported that roughly one third of top firearm shooters mentally rehearsed out of their eyes, another third used the third person method, and the last third used both.

Try them both to see if you have a preference. If you like both, use first person one day and third person the next. Studies show both are effective.

Confidence Improvement

So many new martial arts students have told me they wanted to develop greater confidence. Confidence is paramount for new soldiers and rookie cops too. We're talking real confidence based on real skills, not confidence based on the authority of the badge, color of the belt, and rank insignia on the uniform. False confidence is worse than having none.

Consistent physical practice combined with mental rehearsal gives you the confidence needed to train, compete, and do your duties to the best of your abilities.

Consider this finding From *Force Science News*, (2013:)

"After an initial shooting exercise to establish a baseline, some officers were exposed to a seven-minute session during which they imagined themselves shooting with unfailing accuracy even when under the stress of an attack, while a control group merely listened to unrelated audio input.

"When then exposed to a simulated gun battle, the mental imagers consistently out-performed the others, whose targeting skills under fire tended to erode significantly from their normal level of accuracy.

"This finding has led the researchers to recommend that imagery exercises not only be incorporated into 'regular' police training and practice but that officers 'use mental imagery whenever they have a spare moment' to improve their performance in what may be life-or-death situations."

Taste

Throughout this book, I remind you to use all five of your senses when imaging. Some people, however, find taste to be the hardest to create in their mind. It needn't be.

The types of tastes and the number of tastes are slightly different throughout the world. I like the Chinese list: sour, sweet, salty, spicy, and bitter. If you have others, feel free to add them.

When you mentally rehearse, you can incorporate the taste of gunpowder, vehicle exhaust, a lasting taste from your most recent meal, chewing gum, cough drop, cigarette, toothpaste, chewing tobacco, blood, and whatever else is indigenous to you and your rehearsed scenario.

A Study Of Cops Who Have Employed Deadly Force

A study by Dr. Darrell Ross, Chairman of the Department of Law Enforcement and Justice Administration at Western Illinois University, looked at 121 male police officers from 94 agencies who were forced to kill suspects. One of the influences Dr. Ross found that predisposed the positive outcomes of deadly force encounters was that officers had formulated a plan, usually on the way to a hot call. Some had mentally rehearsed similar situations far in advance.

Dr. Ross's study found about one third of the 121 officers had formal training in mental rehearsal and many others had practiced it on their own, probably having learned from books, videos, and seminars.

All of the officers had benefitted to some degree by mentally preparing for the danger they were about to encounter. In short, they used performance rehearsal to increase their awareness and ready their responses.

War Story

There were seven Plaid Pantries, 7-11s, and other mini markets in my beat and each week one or two of them were robbed at gunpoint during my patrol shift. One year, about a week before Christmas, all seven were robbed the same night. Most cops agree an armed robbery is a highly dangerous call because the suspects are desperate, often drug addicts, and willing to risk all for $40.

Although I had lots of experience responding to hold-ups and I thought I followed good tactics, I wanted to respond more smoothly, as if I had physically practiced at each of the seven stores.

Enter mental rehearsal.

Because literally practicing at the stores was out of the question, I did the next best thing. Whenever I wasn't on a call, I would park across the street from one of the properties and study the layout, and consider such possibilities as:

- the volume of customers, inside and outside at different times of the day.
- the number of approaches to the store.
- the many avenues of escape.
- what I could see through the store's windows.
- the location of the cash register.
- the best approach if the crook was still inside.
- at what point he could see me.
- what the backdrop was should he engage me with his weapon.
- where I would position my backup.

There were always variations too.

- the suspect was still on the premises; the suspect had already fled.
- dispatch gave me the direction of his escape; his direction of escape was unknown.
- dispatch said the suspect was still on the premises; dispatch didn't know if he was there.

Once I picked a variation, I would practice one of two types of mental rehearsal:

- If I were parked where there were lots of passersby looking at me, I would take a couple of deep breaths, keep my eyes open, and proceed to rehearse.
- If no one could see in the car, I would use one of the calming methods described in the last section to better embed my mental rehearsal in my mind. But since I was working, I kept my eyes open and didn't go as deeply as I would if I were doing it at home.

Understand that while this might sound like a lot to do, especially when you're working, the entire process plays out in as little as 30 seconds. So in 2 ½ minutes, I practiced my tactics 5 times.

If time was limited, I mentally rehearsed just one scenario, say, one in which 1) I encountered the holdup man leaving the store; 2) it was dark; 3) there were lots of people around. That is three elements, but enough to make for an interesting scenario.

After just a few sessions, I found myself responding to subsequent hold-up calls more smoothly and confidently than I had previously.

All because I had practiced, albeit only in my mind.

Keep At It

You don't expect to build bulging biceps after one barbell curl so don't expect results with mental rehearsal after one session. That said, results come much faster with mental rehearsal than with lifting weights. Additionally, it's a lot easier and you don't have to drive to a gym.

The gym is in your head, wherever you are.

CHAPTER 9

MENTAL REHEARSAL METHODS

Use the following mental rehearsal methods as is or as a guide to creating your own for your specific needs. Don't let the thought of making your own intimidate you. It's hard to mess this up. Simply apply these elements and you're good to go.

- Determine what you want to rehearse: training technique, kata, technique maintenance, shooting skill, hand-to-hand fighting, gunfight, dangerous vehicle stop, violent arrest, crowd control, public speech, oral test, arguing your case, and so on.
- Choose a meditation technique you like.
- Whether the real action takes two minutes to do physically or only five seconds, your mental rehearsal should take the same amount of time.
- Rehearse with all your senses. Feel it, see it, smell it, hear it, and taste it.
- Be prepared for great results.

Within each mental rehearsal method you're given three time periods from which to choose. Because each one serves a different purpose, you're encouraged to become knowledgeable with all three. They are:

- Quick Session: 2 to 5 minutes
- Mini Movements: 10 to 15 minutes
- Deep Meditation: 20 to 30 minutes

MENTAL REHEARSAL 1: FOR CALMNESS

Martial artists, cops, and soldiers know the importance of remaining calm in the face of a threat. An agitated mind, fearful mind, and an enraged mind can quickly deteriorate, debilitate, and even negate all your hard training. Indeed, learning to remain calm when everyone else is frantic gives you a powerful advantage before the battle starts, during it, and after it ends.

Some actors jog in place or hammer their chests with their fists to amp up their energy before a scene; some weight lifters scream and slap their faces before a heavy lift; I knew cops who listened to "Flight of the Valkyries" (from the movie *Apocalypse Now*) before serving a high-risk warrant; and some soldiers in Afghanistan listen to loud, slamming music when heading out on a mission.

While the above methods and others are important to psyche up before engaging in a stressful event, there are times when being calm is equally important before, during, and after. I'll leave it to you to decide where each applies in your life.

For now, let's get calm.

Quick Session: 2 To 5 Minutes

- You're sitting in your squad car after having just wrestled a violent subject into booking.
- You're a brown belt martial artist and your instructor just told you to spar Bruno, a black belt of exemplary skill.
- You were notified to report to the First Sergeant right away to explain your actions at the base bar last night.

The bad news is you've got only minutes to get yourself calm and collected. The good news is you got Quick Session.

- If possible, find a place to be alone for a few minutes. If this is impossible, sit or stand calmly wherever you might be.
- Think or whisper your trigger word and feel the first wave of calmness wash over your body, from your head to your toes. Think or whisper it two or three times, enjoying each subsequent sensation of calmness and relaxation.
- Now, inhale slowly and follow your breath as it enters your nose, travels down your throat and chest, and expands your lower belly.
- Exhale slowly and feel it leave your lower belly, travel up through your chest and throat, and exit silently out of your mouth.
- Each time you exhale, think or whisper "calm," "relax," or whatever word connotes to you a quiet, tranquil mind.
- Repeat the inhalation and exhalation procedure two more times. If you have time to repeat it four or fives times, do so.

Hold onto that wonderful sense of mental calm and physical relaxation as you begin to mentally rehearse.

- Feel your body relax. Image the muscles in your neck, shoulders, and torso becoming heavy. Feel the same in your rear, legs and feet.
- Smell something pleasant, even if you have to draw upon a memory. Maybe it's the smell of popcorn or a mountain lake.
- See the lake undisturbed and ripple free.
- Taste the fresh mountain air.
- Repeat this procedure as many times as your time allotment allows.

- When the time is up, tell yourself you will continue to feel this powerful sense of calm as you proceed with whatever awaits you in the next few minutes.

Key Points

- In the other Quick Sessions that follow, you will practice your activity a few times. With this one, you're using your limited time just to calm your mind and body.
- Use all your senses for as long as your session allows. Allow these things to calm your mind, slow your heart rate, and remove tension from your muscles.
- Strive to deepen the sensation you felt from your trigger word as you begin to focus on your breathing. Then as you proceed through your five senses, try to deepen your sense of calm and relaxation even more.

Mini Movements: 10 To 15 Minutes

Compared to some of the other mini movement scenarios that follow, there isn't as much to do when imaging calmness. I suppose you could pantomime sipping an adult beverage in the shade of a Hawaiian palm tree, but don't.

Instead, mentally rehearse small movements as if adjusting your body into a place of comfort and total relaxation.

Let's use the same setup as in Quick Session. You're a cop trying to mellow out after a scuffle; you're a brown belt getting ready to spar a tough black belt; or you're about to talk to the First Sergeant about your poor decisions the night before.

For the meditation phase, let's use the breathing technique as described above in "Sitting Meditation 1: Basic follow your breath meditation."

- If possible, find a place to be alone for a few minutes. If this is impossible, sit or stand calmly wherever you might be.
- Think or whisper your trigger word. Feel the first wave of calmness wash over your body, from your head to your toes. Think or whisper it two or three times, enjoying the sensation of calmness and relaxation wash over you.
- Now, inhale slowly and follow your breath as it enters your nose, travels down your throat and chest, and expands your lower belly.

- Exhale slowly as you feel it leave your lower belly, travel up through your chest and throat, and exit silently out your mouth.
- Each time you exhale, think or whisper "calm," "relax," or whatever words connotes to you a quiet, tranquil mind.
- Repeat the inhalation and exhalation procedure for the next several minutes.

Now, hold onto that wonderful sense of mental calm and physical relaxation as you begin to apply mini movements.

- Inhale slowly and deeply, filling your belly.
- As you slowly exhale, wiggle your body a little to settle into your deep relaxation. Feel a sense of calm wash over you.
- Inhale slowly and deeply, filling your belly.
- Exhale *sharply*, as if you plopped into your favorite chair at the end of an exhausting day. Feel a wave of relaxation and gentle calm wash over you.
- Inhale slowly and deeply, filling your belly.
- Lift your arms just a little. As you slowly exhale, let your arms plop back down to where they were, as if all your arm and shoulder muscles suddenly dissolved. Feel a sense of calm wash over you.
- Inhale slowly and deeply, filling your belly.
- As you slowly exhale, allow your face muscles to go slack, and your mouth to drop open. Feel a powerful sense of calm wash over you.
- Repeat this procedure as many times as you can.
- When the time is up, tell yourself you will continue to feel this powerful sense of calm as you proceed with your day.

Key Points

- In later mental imagery exercises, you learn to mentally rehearse fighting the black belt and talking to the sergeant. The above method is about instilling calm and relaxation.
- With each mini movement it's important to image the calm and relaxation you want.
- Feel it in your muscles, abdomen, shoulders, and face.
- Feel your mind become as calm as a still lake, void of ripples and debris.

Deep Meditation: 20 To 30 Minutes

As a martial artist, you might get to your school early and do deep meditation in your car or in an empty room in your school.

As a cop, you might do this in a back room at the station or in your car before you hit the street.

As a soldier, do this anywhere you won't be disturbed.

Follow your breath as described above in "Quick Session" and "Mini Movements," but do it for 10 or 15 minutes to go as deeply as you're able. You can alternate the time, say, 10 minutes for meditation and 15 minutes for mental rehearsal. Next time, meditate for 15 minutes and follow with 10 minutes of mental rehearsal.

- If possible, find a place to be alone or a corner to be by yourself for a few minutes. If this is impossible, sit or stand calmly wherever you might be.
- Think or whisper your trigger word. Feel the first wave of calmness wash over your body, from your head to your toes. Think or whisper it two or three times, enjoying the sensation of calmness and relaxation.
- Now, inhale slowly and follow your breath as it enters your nose, travels down your throat and chest, and expands your lower belly.
- Exhale slowly as you feel it leave your lower belly, travel up through your chest and throat, and exit silently out your mouth.
- Each time you exhale, think or whisper "calm," "relax," or whatever words connotes to you a quiet, tranquil mind.
- Repeat the inhalation and exhalation procedure for the next several minutes.

Now you're calm, relaxed, and receptive to your mental rehearsal. There are many ways to image calmness, but the most popular is to conjure a time in your life when you were at your most mellow. That ultra relaxing weekend at the beach; floating on a water mattress on a summer lake; slumping in your easy chair in front of the tube; or listening to a string concerto while sitting in the dark. (If you're a Marine Gunney and your most mellow moment is lying in a bubble-filled bath with candles all around, best to keep it to yourself.)

For our purposes, let's say you're sprawled on a chaise lounge at the beach.

- Feel the comfortable, soothing warmth of the sun on your body. Feel it from your face to your feet. Feel how the gentle breeze caresses your body.
- Hear the sounds of seagulls overhead and the crash of waves.
- Smell the salty air.
- See the rhythm of the crystal clear, undulating waves, and the clear-blue sky.
- Taste the salt in the air.
- For several minutes, allow your mind to experience these senses. Experience one at a time, two or more at a time, or all five at the same time. Allow your imagery to bring peace and calm to your mind and body.
- When the time is up, tell yourself you will continue to feel this powerful sense of calm as you proceed with your day.

Key Points

- There is a difference between doing things you enjoy—shooting, kata, defensive tactics—and doing things that deeply relax you and make you feel at peace. It's the latter you want to bring to your mental rehearsal.
- Just before you conclude your mental rehearsal practice, a time when you're deeply calm and your subconscious is highly suggestive, take a moment to reinforce your trigger word. Tell yourself, "Whenever I whisper or think _____ [insert your trigger word], I feel a deep sense of calm and relaxation." Think or whisper this to yourself several times before you end your session.

MENTAL REHEARSAL 2: FACING AN ADVERSARY

Adversaries: foreign enemy, police suspect, martial arts competitor, mugger, coworker, you name it. For our purposes here, the adversary has not become violent, though there is an air of threat about him. Often, your calm demeanor will quell the person and situation before it can escalate.

To respond at your optimum requires you to be in control of yourself and, as much as possible, the situation. Boxing champ Mike Tyson said:

"I'm scared every time I go into the ring, but it's how you handle it. What you have to do is plant your feet, bite down on your mouthpiece and say, Let's go."

You must also be *mentally prepared*. Here is what Muhammad Ali said:

"Champions aren't made in gyms. Champions are made from something they have deep inside them—a desire, a dream, a vision. They have to have last-minute stamina; they have to be a little faster; and they have to have the skill and the will. But the will must be stronger than the skill."

A strong will to prevail in the face of adversity is a potent weapon. When it's supplemented with powerful mental rehearsal and well-polished physical skills, you become a force to reckon with.

For our purpose here, let's make the adversary a coworker or a fellow trainee.

Quick Session: 2 To 5 Minutes

- Find a place to be alone for a few minutes. If this is impossible, sit or stand calmly wherever you might be.
- Think or whisper your trigger word. Feel the first wave of calmness wash over your body, from your head to your toes. Think or whisper it two or three times, enjoying the sensation of calmness and relaxation envelop your body.
- Inhale slowly, mentally following your breath as it enters through your nose, travels down your throat and chest, and expands your lower belly.
- Exhale slowly, mentally following it as it leaves your lower belly, travels up through your chest and throat, and exits silently out your mouth.

The above procedure takes one to two minutes to prepare your mind. Use the following mental rehearsal procedure as is, or tweak it to fit your specific need.

- See the person in your mind. Make this image as clear and detail-rich as you're able: the setting, the adversary's physical appearance, and the situation in which you make contact.
- Hear, smell and taste the setting where you're likely to face him: factory, shooting range, city street, office, school, or base of operations.
- Feel a strong sense of relaxation throughout your body. Feel your demeanor as calm and cool.
- See and feel the adversary's negative demeanor as he speaks to you.
- Feel yourself remain calm and cool no matter what he says or how he acts.
- See yourself standing tall and poised in the face of the person's words and demeanor.
- Hear yourself speak calmly and with control.
- If you know what you're going to say, hear the words in your mind. Hear how calmly you're saying them and articulately you're uttering the words.
- Repeat the process as many times as you can in the time allotment.
- When the time is up, tell yourself you will continue to feel this powerful sense of calm and confidence as you proceed with your day.

Key Points

- Do a Quick Session as often as you're able. If possible, do it right before contact with the person. The more you practice, the better you will respond in reality.

Mini Movements: 10 To 15 Minutes

For this session, let's use "Sitting Meditation 2: Four-Part Breath" as described earlier. It's an easy-to-do breathing technique guaranteed to instill calm and relaxation. It works whether you're standing or sitting.

- Make whatever adjustments to your stance or seated position to get comfortable.
- Think or whisper your trigger word two or three times
- Take two or three slow breath exchanges to settle your body and alert your brain as to what you're about to do.
- Tell yourself you're going to follow your breath for a few minutes to bring on an enjoyable sense of calm to your mind and body.

Now you're ready to begin 4-part breathing pattern.

- As you inhale through your nose, feel the oxygen slowly expand your lower belly.
- Then slowly expand your ribs.
- Then slowly expand your chest.
- Then feel the air in your throat.

Hold for 5 to 10 seconds. Don't strain. Now reverse the process, exhaling out your mouth.

- Feel the air slowly leave your throat.
- Then slowly leave your chest.
- Then slowly leave your rib area.
- Then slowly deflate your belly.
- Repeat this breathing pattern for five or 10 minutes.

You're now ready to commence with mental rehearsal and mini movements.

- See the adversary in front of you, using as much detail as possible.
- If he normally fills you with anxiety, don't show it. Feel how calm you are, how relaxed you are, and how confident you are in his presence.
- Whether you're standing or sitting, use mini movements to straighten your posture, lengthen your spine, and look him straight in the eyes.
- Use mini movements to depict holding your hands close to your chest, palms open toward the adversary. (Psychologists say this can have a calming effect on some hostile people. Some, not all.)
- Whisper or think your diffusing verbal response to him.
- Feel how calm you are. Feel it in your body and in your mind.
- Use mini movements to depict walking away from him.
- Turn your head slightly to mimic watching him in your peripheral.
- Repeat your mental rehearsal as many times as you can. If there are other details not listed here, add them. Be sure to include all your senses.
- When the time is up, tell yourself you will continue to feel this powerful sense of calm and confidence as you proceed with your day.

Key Points

- Add additional movements as they apply to you and your situation. If the adversary has approached you while you're dressing for training, use mini movements to mimic putting on your clothes, all the while staying calm and confident. If he gets in your face at work, use mini movements to depict what you do on your job. Through it all, mentally rehearsal a calm and relaxed demeanor.

Deep Meditation: 20 To 30 Minutes

Use the "Sitting Meditation 2: Four-Part Breath" as just described in "Mini Movements." Do this seated or standing.

- Make whatever adjustments to your stance or seated position to get comfortable.
- Think or whisper your trigger word two or three times

- Take two or three slow breaths exchanges to settle your body and alert your brain as to what you're about to do.
- Tell yourself you're going to follow your breath for a few minutes to bring on an enjoyable sense of calm to your mind and body.

Now you're ready to begin the 4-part breathing pattern.

- As you inhale through your nose, feel the oxygen slowly expand your lower belly.
- Then slowly expand your ribs.
- Then slowly expand your chest.
- Then feel the air in your throat.

Hold for 5 to 10 seconds. Don't strain. Now reverse the process out your mouth.

- Feel the air slowly leave your throat.
- Then slowly leave your chest.
- Then slowly leave your rib area.
- Then slowly deflate your belly.
- Repeat this breathing pattern for five or 10 minutes.

Take as long as you want to get as deeply calm and relaxed as you're able. The more sedate your mind, the more receptive it is to positive mental rehearsal.

Now you're ready to proceed with mental rehearsal.

- Hear, smell, feel, and taste the environment where you're likely to contact the adversary Strive to make everything real in your mind.
- See every detail of him. If he scowls, see it. If he has a fake smile, see it.
- Hear him speak with as much detail as you're able. If doing so fills you with anxiety, take a moment to slowly and deeply inhale into your belly, and then slowly exhale it. Do this repeatedly, and each time feel a sense of calm replace your anxiety.
- See and feel your posture straighten, your body relax, and your gaze fall on the adversary. Feel your face relaxed and without expression.

- Hear what you would say to him. Hear your tone void of fear, anxiety, and of antagonism. Hear your carefully chosen deescalating words.
- Every minute or so, think or whisper your trigger word to cloak yourself with calm.
- Repeat the mental rehearsal as many times as you can in the time you have allotted.
- When the time is up, tell yourself you will continue to feel this powerful sense of calm and confidence as you proceed with your day.

Key Points

- After repeating the mental rehearsal two or three times, it's okay if you want to add mini movements to this session.

MENTAL REHEARSAL 3: HIGH-RISK VEHICLE STOP

A vehicle that has been stopped for a routine check by the military or for a traffic violation by the police involves an element of the unknown. The occupant could very well be a law abiding person, someone who has just committed a violent crime, a wanted criminal, a person wired with explosives, or someone who wants to kill a police officer or an American soldier.

The stop might be yet another checkpoint or another traffic violation but cops and soldiers must always be mentally prepared for any possibility. Indeed, the term "routine traffic stop" needs to be removed from the vernacular and the mindset of police officers and the military.

Quick Session: 2 To 5 Minutes

If your job involves frequent car stops, you should do a Quick Session at least once a day.

- Find a place to be alone for a few minutes. If this is impossible, sit or stand calmly wherever you might be.
- Think or whisper your trigger word. Feel the first wave of calmness wash over your body, from your head to your toes. Think or whisper it two or three times, enjoying the sensation of calmness and relaxation envelop your body.
- Inhale slowly, mentally following your breath as it enters through your nose, travels down your throat and chest, and expands your lower belly.
- Exhale slowly, mentally following it leave your lower belly, travel up through your chest and throat, and exit silently out your mouth.
- Follow your breath for a full minute or two, allowing it to calm you as much as possible in the minimum time period.

A tad calmer now, you're ready to practice mental rehearsal.

- See whatever is outside your windshield: the hood of your vehicle, traffic moving in the same direction as you, oncoming traffic, street signs, and streetlights.
- Hear your radio, smell the interior, feel the steering wheel, and taste what you normally taste.
- See the vehicle you're going to stop or approach.
- Think or whisper your trigger word and feel it calm you.
- Mentally rehearse with all your senses what you would do: hear your words as you inform dispatch; see your hand activate your overhead lights; see the driver and passengers react; see your hands steer your vehicle behind the target vehicle, hear yours or your partner's commands over the PA system.
- Think or whisper your trigger word and feel it calm you.
- Tell yourself you're in control of youself and the situation. You're alert to any sudden movement and you're ready to take whatever action is necessary should things suddenly deteriorate.
- Repeat as many times as you can.
- When the time is up, tell yourself you will continue to feel this

powerful sense of calm and confidence as you proceed with your day.

Key Points

- Please keep in mind that in practice, the actual Quick Session takes far less time than it does to read the above description. Once you get into the habit of doing them, they get easier and the results come faster.

Mini Movements: 10 To 15 Minutes

For "Mini Movements," let's kick up the intensity a notch and say you're in a patrol car or military vehicle and you have pulled behind a pickup in which there is an armed and dangerous man.

While you can choose any meditation method you want from Section 2 to establish deep calm and relaxation, let's say you have only 10 minutes to practice mini movements. So you've decided to bring on a mild sense of calm using only your trigger word as described earlier in the subsection "Create a Trigger Word." As noted, when implemented correctly a trigger word can be used to bring on a mild sense of calm and relaxation, to jumpstart a meditation method, or to reestablish the meditative state when something has disturbed your session.

- Get comfortable in your standing or seated position.
- Take a slow, deep inhalation into your belly. Feel it there and see it there. (Some meditators like to image the air as a cool, aqua blue color.) As you slowly exhale, see it leave your belly, travel up your chest, pass through your throat, and out your mouth.
- Every time you exhale, think or whisper your trigger word twice. As you do, image your body and mind becoming relaxed and calm. Repeat as many times as you like. If you only have 10 minutes for everything, do it for 4 or 5 minutes.

You're now ready to mentally rehearse and use mini movements. Remember, mini movements are, well, mini. You don't have to extend your arms all the way out or turn your body 180 degrees. Moving two or three inches is sufficient, whether extending, turning, ducking, or kicking.

- Use all your senses to image yourself in your vehicle. See what you normally see; hear what you normally hear; smell what you normally smell; feel what you normally feel; and taste what you normally taste.
- You and your partner see the dirty white pickup parked on a dark, dead-end street. Move your face forward a little and squint as if you're alerting on the vehicle and checking the license plate. It's midnight and the truck's interior and exterior lights are off.
- Tilt your head a little to the right to hear your partner call in your location to dispatch. Say aloud or think a brief discussion with your partner about how to proceed.
- Using mini motions with your arms and legs, open the driver's door and step out. If you're seated, do the mini motions but imagine yourself standing. Feel the gravel under your feet and duck your head a little as if taking cover behind your door. Hear your partner get out and hear him tell the driver to get out. Use a mini motion to mimic gripping the butt of your holstered weapon.
- Crouch a little lower as you hear and see the pickup driver's door open. See his left leg start to get out, then stop. Hear your partner tell him to show his hands. See him refuse.
- Feel adrenaline surge through your body and use a mini movement to draw your weapon. Use a mini motion to bring it up and look over the barrel at the suspect still sitting in his truck.
- See the driver step out quickly—white male, 30s, tall, white T-shirt, blue jeans—and turn toward you. Mini crouch, and see him in your harsh headlights and spotlight.
- See him lift the handgun, the end of its barrel pointing at you. Whisper or think "Gun!" Hear your partner shout, "Drop the weapon!"
- Hear and see the whitish/orangish explosions from his gun. Hear your gun and your partner's. Use small movements with your hand to duplicate your weapon's slight recoil.
- Hear the sound of breaking glass to your right and hear glass spray across the seats inside your vehicle.
- Continue to use a mini motion to extend your weapon as you see the suspect slam back against his truck door. See him drop his weapon and curl down to the gravel.
- Smell and taste the gun smoke now. Feel your heart racing. Hear your partner shouting commands at the downed suspect.

- Repeat the mental rehearsal scenario as often as your time allows.
- When the time is up, tell yourself you will continue to feel alert, energized, but calm and confident as you proceed with your day.

Key Points

- Although mini movements are fractional, they are complete movements in your mind. You might find that closing your eyes or partially closing them to blur your vision helps you mentally rehearse better.
- Use your senses as you move. Feel the door you push open; taste the gun smoke you see wafting through the air; hear the whine of the bullet.

Deep Meditation: 20 To 30 Minutes

For this session, let's use your trigger word and the breathing method described in "Sitting Meditation 1: Basic Follow Your Breath Meditation" together before practicing mental rehearsal.

Use the same situation as described above. You're in a patrol car or military vehicle and you have pulled behind a pickup in which there is an armed and dangerous man. The primary difference between this method and mini movements is this time you're not moving, which means all the action plays out in your mind.

- Get comfortable in your standing or seated position.
- Take a slow, deep inhalation into your belly. Feel it there and see it there.
- As you slowly exhale, see it leave your belly, travel up your chest, pass through your throat, and out your mouth.
- Think or whisper your trigger word twice, and feel your body and mind becoming relaxed and calm.
- Then take another slow, deep inhalation into your belly. Feel it there and see it there.
- As you slowly exhale, see it leave your belly, travel up your chest, pass through your throat, and out your mouth.
- Again, think or whisper your trigger word twice, and feel your body and mind becoming relaxed and calm.
- Repeat this process for at least 10 minutes.

- Once you're tranquil and cloaked in a wonderful feeling of relaxation, take a minute or two to enjoy the sensation.

Now you're ready to practice mental rehearsal.

- Use all your senses to image yourself in your vehicle. See what you normally see; hear what you normally hear; smell what you normally smell; feel what you normally feel; and taste what you normally taste.
- See the dirty white pickup parked on a dead end street in an area in which there are no other people. It's midnight and the truck's lights, interior and exterior are off. You have a partner. Smell the interior of your vehicle. Feel the steering wheel in your hands.
- See your partner pick up the mic. Hear him call in your location. Hear you and your partner discuss your approach.
- See and feel yourself open the driver's door and step out. Hear your partner get out as he continues to tell the driver of the suspicious vehicle to get out. Feel the gravel under your feet and see the open door in front as you crouch behind it. (If you have angled your car enough, see yourself crouched behind the trunk or the hood.)
- See and hear the driver's door open. See his left leg start to get out, then stop.
- Hear your partner tell him to show his hands. He doesn't do it.
- Feel adrenaline surge through your body as you draw your weapon. See and feel yourself bring it up and look over the barrel at the suspect still sitting in his truck.
- See the driver—white male, 30s, tall, white T-shirt, blue jeans—step quickly from the vehicle and turn toward you. See how well illuminated he is in your vehicle's harsh headlights and spotlight.
- See him lift the handgun, the end of its barrel pointing at you. Hear yourself shout "Gun!" Hear your partner shout, "Drop the weapon!"
- See flashes from his gun. Hear your gun explode and feel its vibration in your hand.
- Hear the sound of breaking glass to your right and hear glass spray inside your vehicle.
- Hear your partner's gun fire round after round and feel your gun bucking in your hand.
- See the suspect slam back against his truck door. See him drop

the weapon as he curls down to the gravel.
- Smell and taste the gun smoke now. Feel your heart racing. Hear your partner shouting commands at the downed suspect.
- Repeat the mental rehearsal as often as your time allows.
- When the time is up, tell yourself you will carry your mental training with you as you proceed with your day.

Key Points

- Modify your mental rehearsal to fit your potential situation: location, time of day, without a partner, on foot instead of in a vehicle, and so on.
- You never get used to being shot at but with good, solid mental rehearsal practice, you might prevent such negative reactions as freezing, indecision, and lack of fire control, such as spray and pray.

MENTAL REHEARSAL 4: LEARNING A NEW SKILL

First, a word about negativity.

Some people are quick to convince themselves they will never be good. "I'm a terrible shooter." "Everyone beats me at sparring." "I never remember law statutes." "I'm a terrible leader."

As long as they think, image, and say these things, they will be right. Studies show—*The Achievement Zone*, Shane Murphy, Berkley Trade, (1997)—negative imagery to be more powerful than positive. But powerful positive imagery in time will replace it. Consider Henry Ford's old adage: "Whether you think you can or whether you think you can't, you're right."

Your task through positive mental rehearsal is to cover up or replace all that negative input you have acquired over the years.

War Story

I was a range officer for a few years. One year we were introducing a new shotgun course in which we would shoot over car hoods, through mock city windows, and skip shoot under cars. One officer in particular, who was otherwise outstanding at her job, had a deathly fear of shotguns. She told me in a trembling voice she had not slept for the past couple of nights knowing she would have to shoot it. I smooth-talked her, explained every element of the course and, I thought, convinced her she would ace the thing. Still shaky as a fall leaf, she loaded the shotgun, took a deep breath, chambered a round, and fired it into the ground 12 inches from my foot. Before I could complete my little girl scream, she discharged another round, missing my foot again by mere inches.

I don't know if she ever finished the course because I left the range for a long break.

This officer was a clear example of how negative thinking can affect your actions.

Note: The below methods describe ways to augment and imbed the instruction into your mind. However, if you're apprehensive about upcoming training, use the meditation and mental rehearsal method as described in "Mental Rehearsal 1: Mental Imagery For Calmness." Image yourself as calm, relaxed, and receptive to the new learning. Be sure to use positive mental rehearsal and positive verbiage. Practice "Quick Session, Mini-Movements," and "Deep Meditation," as often as you can each day leading up to the instruction.

Here is another Henry Ford Quote: "One of the greatest discoveries a man makes, one of his greatest surprises, is to find he can do what he was afraid he couldn't do."

Let's make the new skill a chest slap to distract followed by a shoulder spin to get behind the adversary.

Quick Session: 2 To 5 Minutes

- Find a place to be alone for a few minutes. If this is impossible, sit or stand calmly wherever you might be.
- Think or whisper your trigger word. Feel the first wave of calmness wash over your body, from your face to your toes. Think or whisper it two or three times, enjoying the sensation envelop your body.
- Inhale slowly, mentally following your breath as it enters through your nose, travels down your throat and chest, and expands your lower belly.
- Exhale slowly, mentally following your breath as it leaves your lower belly, travels up through your chest and throat, and exits silently out your mouth.

You're now ready to mentally rehearse the slap and spin.

- See the adversary in front of you. See his demeanor as antagonistic, threatening, and hostile. Hear his threats, feel your adrenaline charge your muscles, and smell and taste the environment you're in.
- See and feel your lead arm lash out without telegraphing and feel your palm slap his upper chest. Hear it land with a loud *Smack!*
- Feel the impact on your hand. See the startled look on his face.
- See and feel the hand you slapped with grab his closest shoulder and see and feel your other hand press his farthest one.
- See and feel your closest hand pull his shoulder and your other hand push the other.
- See and feel him turn as you simultaneously step behind him.
- Repeat the mental rehearsal as often as your time allows.
- When the time is up, tell yourself you will carry your new technique with you as you proceed with your day.

Key Points

- The entire technique will take you six seconds to mentally rehearse. This means you can do as many as 60 reps!
- Add whatever follow-up you want: pull him down, wrap your arm around his neck for a sleeper hold, or run away.

Mini Movements: 10 To 15 Minutes

Be careful where you do these. Martial artists will have an easier time practicing mini movements around their peers than cops and soldiers. In the mid 1970s when the martial arts were still relatively new in the United States, I got dispatched to a mental subject flopping around in a park. When I got there, I found a man—a completely sane one—simply practicing a kata. So until everyone learns and accepts the power of mini movements, choose wisely where you do them.

For "Mini Movements" and "Deep Meditation" that follows, let's use "Sitting Meditation 5: 8-count breathing." As mentioned when introduced earlier, you might experience a small learning curve when doing 8-count. If you tried 4-count discussed in *Meditation for Warriors*, you probably took to it easily. With this one, however, each stage takes twice as long. You might get it the first time or it might take you a few tries to determine how much air to take in and to release. It's definitely worth the effort.

- Get comfortable wherever you're sitting. Scoot a little this way and that way and wiggle your butt to get your sit-down muscles where you want them.
- Think or whisper your trigger word three times
- Take two or three deep breaths to settle your body and alert your brain as to what you're about to do.

You're now ready to commence the meditation phase.

- Breathe in slowly through your nose to a count of 8: 1, 2, 3, 4, 5, 6, 7, 8.
- Hold it in for a count of 8: 1, 2, 3, 4, 5, 6, 7, 8.
- Exhale out your mouth for a count of 8: 1, 2, 3, 4, 5, 6, 7, 8.
- Hold it for a count of 8: 1, 2, 3, 4, 5, 6, 7, 8.
- Repeat the cycle for as many times as you like to get as mentally calm and physically relaxed as you can.

Now you're ready to do mini movements. Whether standing or sitting, move your arms, legs and body minimally to simulate full movements

- See the adversary in front of you, his demeanor as antagonistic, threatening, and hostile.

- Turn your body slightly to blade yourself. Lift your hands a little to simulate raising your arms, hands palms forward, and close to your chest.
- Make your face neutral and look forward (even if your eyes are closed) as if looking at his face. See all of his body in your peripheral. Hear his threats, feel adrenaline charge your muscles, and smell and taste the environment you're in.
- Use a mini movement to lash out with your lead palm to slap his upper chest.
- Hear it land with a loud *Smack!* Feel the impact and see the startled look on his face.
- Use a mini movement with the same hand you slapped with to duplicate grabbing his closest shoulder. Use a mini movement with your other hand to press his farthest one.
- Use mini movements to pull his closest shoulder and push his farthest one.
- See and feel him turn as you use mini movements to twist him about.
- Use mini movements with your legs to simulate stepping behind him.
- Repeat this mini movement stage as many times as you like. Always strive to use all your senses and to mentally rehearse every stage as clearly as possible.
- When the time is up, tell yourself you will carry your newly imbedded skill with you as you proceed with your day.

Key Points

- I deliberately stopped the technique description with you standing behind the person and your body flush with his backside. If your instructor included a follow-up, go ahead and add that to your mental rehearsal.
- Keep in mind that reading the procedure takes much longer that imaging. Imaging it takes 4 to 6 seconds.

Deep Meditation: 20 To 30 Minutes

Now let's deeply embed the chest slap and shoulder twist. If the technique is new to you, do meditation and mental rehearsal daily until you have it down (it won't take long before you do). If you learned it last class and today your instructor is going to see how well you do it, practice your meditation and mental rehearsal before your training. If you have a choice, do it first thing after waking up when your mind is relaxed and susceptible to your input.

- Get comfortable wherever you're sitting. Scoot a little this way and that way and wiggle your butt to get your sit-down muscles where you want them.
- Think or whisper your trigger word three times
- Take two or three deep breaths to settle your body and alert your brain as to what you're about to do.

You're now ready to commence the meditation phase. Again use "Sitting Meditation 5: 8-count breathing."

- Breathe in slowly through your nose to a count of 8: 1, 2, 3, 4, 5, 6, 7, 8.
- Hold it in for a count of 8: 1, 2, 3, 4, 5, 6, 7, 8.
- Exhale out your mouth for a count of 8: 1, 2, 3, 4, 5, 6, 7, 8.
- Hold it for a count of 8: 1, 2, 3, 4, 5, 6, 7, 8.
- Repeat the cycle for as many times as you like to get as mentally calm and physically relaxed as you can.

Now you're ready to enhance your skill.

- See the adversary in front of you. See his demeanor as antagonistic, threatening, and hostile. Use the additional time to really see the person and experience any emotion he might conjure in you.
- Hear his threats, feel adrenaline charge your muscles, smell and taste the environment you're in.
- Feel a powerful sense of confidence in your ability to do the technique. You know it; you understand it; now is the time to solidify it into your muscle memory.

- See and feel your lead arm lash out without telegraphing and feel your palm strike his upper chest. Hear it land with a loud *Smack!* You're not trying to hurt the guy, but rather startle him with speed and sound.
- See the startled look on his face. Allow that to charge you with energy.
- See and feel the hand you smacked him with grab his closest shoulder. See your other hand press his farthest one. Feel your muscles prepare to explode.
- See and feel your closest hand pull and your other push with speed, power, and control.
- See and feel him twist about as you simultaneously step behind him. Feel him flush against your front.
- Add any follow-up you might have learned or just practice this entry.
- Repeat the mental rehearsal as often as your time allows.
- When the time is up, tell yourself you know the technique and feel confident with it as you proceed with your day.

Key Points

- The benefit from deep meditation comes from the depth of your meditative state. If at anytime you feel it start to slip away—a loud noise from outside penetrates your skull, your dog licks your face, your cell rings (don't look at it or answer it)—take a moment to whisper or think your trigger word. Or, do two or three minutes of the meditation method you used to return to your meditative state.
- Deep Meditation allows for lots of time. Meditate for 10 minutes and practice mental rehearsal for 15. Or meditate for 15 and do mental rehearsal for 10, 12 or 15 minutes. Do it the same way every time or mix it up each session.

MENTAL REHEARSAL 5: SKILL MAINTENANCE

Let's say you're experiencing a period in your life where you're happy with your skills in a particular area. For our purposes here, let's make it your empty hand fighting techniques, whether military, law enforcement, or martial arts. Let's say you can't train for a while because you've been hurt, you have other obligations, or you need to concentrate in another area of training (be sure to use mental rehearsal for that too).

Mental practice can help you maintain your skill and do so without raising a sweat or getting a bruise.

War Story:

I was a hardcore martial arts tournament competitor in the late 1980s, which is also when I began learning mental rehearsal, or imagery, as we called it then. The Northwest National Karate Tournament was a couple of months away and although I had done well in weapons kata there in the past (with two Japanese sickles called *kama*), I wanted to introduce a new weapon, one used in feudal Japan called *manrikigusari*, a long chain with a weight attached to one end.

Both of these kata were over 100 moves long and both were physically exhausting to perform. Since I was entering other divisions as well, I had only so much energy to train. I saw this as a perfect time to try this thing I was learning—mental imagery, sweatless practice—with the sickles kata.

I physically practiced the chain kata repetitiously nearly every day for over two months. The sickle form, however, I practiced only in my mind. I would image it while I was driving, waiting in line, working a stakeout in my police job, and in the comfort of my easy chair at home. I included all the elements you're learning in this book to image, that is, mentally rehearse, the complete form over and over.

On tournament day, I got a 5th place with the chain kata and won 1st place with the sickles. Then all the first place winners in each division competed for overall grand champion. I won that too. My moment in the sun.

I won my division and overall champion with a 100-movement, technically difficult, and dangerous kata with razor sharp weapons that *I had practiced mentally for two months.*

War Story 2

I know a guy who is a top competitive shooter who at different times has held an assortment of national titles. He shoots for sport and for self-defense. He is a soft-spoken man, intelligent, and pleasant. What sets him apart is this: Virtually everyday as he commutes on a train to and from work, he shoots people. Kinda.

He uses the Quick Session method in which he takes a few slow and deep inhalations and exhalations to relax before choosing his target. It might be someone sitting and reading or someone innocently holding onto a ceiling strap. Once his selection is made, he images sight, smell, touch, hearing, and taste, and zeroes in on his target—sometimes the head and other times center mass—and squeezes his imaginary trigger.

He says it helps his shooting skill and knows it will help him to not hesitate should he ever face a real life and death confrontation.

For this exercise, let's make the technique a defense against a low tackle. Your simple response is to jam the attacker's shoulders with your forearms and sprawl your legs back as you force him to the ground. If you have a different defense, humor me and practice this one until you get the hang of the process. Then feel free to modify the procedure to fit your preferred technique.

Of course, what happens after the takedown depends on your job.

- As a martial artist you would flee, since you've negated the initial attack, or if you deem it necessary, restrain him with a control hold, such as a joint lock.
- As a police officer, you would need to quickly control the attacker using a pain compliance hold and maneuver him into a position to be handcuffed.

- As a soldier defending against an enemy, you would try to control the threat or finish him off with a debilitating or lethal technique.

So the initial defense—shoulder jam, sprawl, and force the attacker to the ground—is the same for everyone. What you do after is up to you and your situation.

Quick Session: 2 To 5 Minutes

- Sit or stand calmly wherever you might be.
- Think or whisper your trigger word and feel the first wave of calmness wash over you, from your head to your toes. Think or whisper it two or three times.
- Now, inhale slowly and follow your breath as it enters your nose, travels down your throat and chest, and expands your lower belly.
- Exhale slowly and feel it silently exit out your mouth.
- Each time you exhale, think or whisper "calm," "relax," or whatever word connotes to you a quiet, tranquil mind.
- Repeat the inhalation and exhalation procedure two more times. If you can do it four or fives times, do so.

Now you're ready to mentally rehearse someone shooting in to tackle you. As a police officer, image the tackle occurring inside of a home in which you've responded to a domestic violence call. As a martial artist, image the tackle on the mat when you're training with a classmate. As a soldier, image a confrontation with a man in your unit.

- See the threat standing in front of you. Hear whatever sounds, smell whatever odors, see whatever people and objects, taste whatever you might taste, and feel whatever you might feel in the environment you're imaging.
- See him shoot toward your legs.
- See, feel, and hear your forearms thump against his shoulders to jam his forward momentum. Feel his energy against your forearms.
- Feel your feet and legs kick back into a sprawl. Feel your feet find purchase.
- Feel your energy drive him down to the floor.

- Hear him grunt as he lands with a splat.
- See and feel yourself flow into your follow-up: flee, control hold, or incapacitate.
- Repeat the mental imagery as often as your time allows.
- When the time is up, tell yourself you know the technique and feel confident with it as you proceed with your day.

Key Points

- Repeat your mental rehearsal in real time for the full two or three minutes. Strive to get in at least a dozen repetitions or more.

Mini Movements: 10 To 15 Minutes

Now you will mentally rehearse your defense against a tackle using small movements that represent your response. Let's use "Sitting Meditation 1: Basic follow your breath meditation," to bring on a deep calm and relaxation.

- Sit or stand calmly wherever you might be.
- Think or whisper your trigger word and feel the first wave of calmness wash over you, from your head to your toes. Think or whisper it two or three times.
- Inhale slowly and follow your breath as it enters your nose, travels down your throat and chest, and expands your lower belly.
- Exhale slowly and feel it leave your lower belly, travel up through your chest and throat, and exit silently out your mouth.
- Each time you exhale, think or whisper "calm," "relax," or whatever words connotes to you a quiet, tranquil mind.
- Repeat the inhalation and exhalation procedure for five to eight minutes. If you can go longer, your meditation will be even deeper.

Now, hold onto this relaxed and calm state as you commence the mini movements, involving as many senses as you can.

- See, hear, feel, smell, and taste all that makes up the imaged environment you're in.

- If you're military, see the threat as a typical soldier or as a specific one. If you're a martial artist, see him as a typical classmate or competitor, or a specific one. If you're a cop, see him as a typical drunken man at a family fight call.
- See him crouch, extend his arms, and launch himself toward you.
- Feel yourself alert on his action: Feel a slight increase in your muscle tension, a slight bend of your upper body, and a slight extension of your arms.
- See him shoot low, his hands inches from wrapping around your hips or upper legs.
- See and feel your upper torso bend forward a little and your legs prepare to spread.
- See your bent arms extend a little more in preparation of slamming your forearms against his shoulders. Feel your energy about to explode into him.
- See and feel your forearms slam his shoulders. Feel the impact in your arms and shoulders and let it jar you and push your arms back a little.
- Feel your feet kick back and actually move them back a few inches. Feel the force of the impact and tense your leg muscles a little.
- See and feel the tackler fall onto his belly or onto all fours.
- Bend over a little as you mentally drive him all the way down. Feel it in your muscles.
- If you're going to step back and draw your weapon, use mini movements to experience all aspects of that motion. If you're going to apply a control hold, mentally rehearse with all of your senses. If you're going to flee, use small motions and all your senses to do so.
- Repeat your mental rehearsal as often as your time allows.
- When the time is up, tell yourself you know the technique and feel confident with it as you proceed with your day.

Key Points

- Some people find imaging the sense of taste difficult. It isn't. You can taste such things as a mint, toothpaste, sweaty atmosphere in a training facility, vehicle exhaust, and dust.
- Besides imaging your body motions, also image any jarring you might feel and the weight and force of your attacker's body.

Deep Meditation: 15 To 25 Minutes

Now let's deeply embed your response to a tackle. Again, use "Sitting Meditation 1: Basic follow your breath meditation," to achieve a meditative state to enable your subconscious to be receptive to your mental rehearsal.

- Find a quiet and comfortable place where you can practice without being disturbed.
- Sit or stand calmly wherever you might be.
- Think or whisper your trigger word and feel the first wave of calmness wash over you, from your head to your toes. Think or whisper it two or three times.
- Inhale slowly and follow your breath as it enters your nose, travels down your throat and chest, and expands your lower belly.
- Exhale slowly and feel it leave your lower belly, travel up through your chest and throat, and exit silently out your mouth.
- Each time you exhale, think or whisper "calm," "relax," or whatever words connotes to you a quiet, tranquil mind.
- Repeat the inhalation and exhalation procedure for 10 minutes or longer. If you can go longer, your meditation will be even deeper.

Now you're calm and relaxed and receptive to your mental rehearsal.

- See him crouch, extend his arms, and launch himself toward you.
- Image yourself solidifying your stance to absorb his impact.
- See him shoot low, his hands inches away from wrapping around your hips or upper legs. Feel his arms encircle your legs.

- See and feel your upper torso bend forward to receive him and your legs begin to spread.
- See and feel your forearms slamming against his shoulders.
- Feel your impact direct his energy downward.
- Feel your feet kick back. Smell his hair.
- See and feel the tackler fall onto his belly or onto his all fours.
- Mentally rehearse holding him down, feel your muscles strain.
- Use all your senses to mentally rehearse your follow-up.
- If you would draw your weapon, rehearse all aspects of that motion. If you're applying a control hold, rehearse it in all your senses. If you're going to flee, rehearse how you would escape.
- Repeat your mental rehearsal as often as your time allows.
- Tell yourself you have progressed and feel confident as you proceed with your day.

Key Points

- You might read the above description of the mental rehearsal procedure and wonder how going through those simple steps could be beneficial. The answer lays in the next to the last bullet: *Repeat your mental rehearsal as often as your time allows.* Benefit comes from repeating the scenario as many times as you can in 10 or 15 minutes in your calm and receptive mind. If you can do it three or four times a minute, that adds up to quite a few reps. Quantity and quality makes the exercise beneficial.
- Your mind will wander when meditating. When it happens, don't sweat it. Simply bring it back to the mental rehearsal and continue. Do the same thing the next time it wanders and again after that. It's the disciplined act of bringing your mind back to your meditation that strengthens your ability to meditate and engage in mental imagery.

MENTAL REHEARSAL 6:

PERFORMANCE ANXIETY DREAMS

In *On Combat*, Lt. Col. Dave Grossman and I wrote about how police officers, even those in elite units, dream about being in a shootout. However, when they return fire, their weapons either jam or miss the target. We wrote that dreams of this type most often occur from a lack of confidence, which usually goes away after the officer practices at a firing range. Since publication of *On Combat*, we have received numerous emails from readers who said their bad dreams stopped after following our advice.

When I was on the PD, and for a few years after, I would dream I was in my patrol car when someone jerked open the door and began pulling me out. I always punched at him but never connected, all the while the threat kept pulling on me. I always woke up before I was all the way extracted. It wasn't until years later when I practiced self-defense in a car for a book, did the dreams stop.

Note: If you're having similar dreams and experiencing them so often they affect your sleep and health, you're strongly advised to seek help from a mental health professional. Also true if you're experiencing dreams from a traumatic event in your past.

Try the following mental rehearsal techniques when you have occasional negative dreams related to your martial arts, police work, or military job. Continue to practice until you achieved results. For some people it might take three or four sessions. Others might require more.

For instructional purposes, let's make the negative dream the one I was having: Someone is trying to pull you out of your personal car, your police unit, or your Humvee.

Quick Session: 2 To 5 Minutes

- Sit or stand calmly wherever you might be.
- Think or whisper your trigger word and feel the first wave of calmness wash over you, from your head to your toes. Think or whisper it two or three times, each time enjoying the sensation of calmness and relaxation.
- Now, inhale slowly and follow your breath as it enters your nose, travels down your throat and chest, and expands your lower belly.
- Exhale slowly as you feel it leave your lower belly, travel up through your chest and throat, and silently exit out your mouth.
- Each time you exhale, think or whisper "calm," "relax," or whatever word connotes to you a quiet, tranquil mind.
- Repeat the inhalation and exhalation procedure two more times. If time allows, do it four or fives times.

Now you're ready to rehearse someone trying to pull you from your vehicle. You're sitting behind the wheel of your parked car on a side street.

- Hear other cars coming and going. Hear a dog barking somewhere.
- Feel the car seat under you and feel your feet on the floor. Feel your hand resting on the top of your steering wheel and the warmth of the sun coming through the window.
- Smell fresh air coming through your partially open window.
- Taste the mint in your mouth.
- See a figure moving toward you out of the corner of your left eye and see him reach for your door handle.
- See and feel yourself twist toward the door.
- See and hear your door jerk open.
- Feel and smell a gush of fresh air wash over you.
- See the man in the door opening. If the threat in your dream is a visible one, image how you dreamt him: race, age, height, weight, and clothing.
- See his arm reach for you. Hear him curse and threaten you.
- Feel your adrenaline surge through your body. Feel the controlled anger fill your head and chest.

- Feel your left hand grab his forearm and feel the tug on your arm as he tries to get his arm back.
- Feel your left foot step out onto the pavement and feel your right leg drive off the floor to propel the rest of you outside.
- Feel your right arm thrust toward the center of his face. Feel your entire body drive your adrenaline-fueled power.
- Feel your palm-heel smash into his nose. Hear his loud grunt of pain.
- Feel your left hand release its grip on his arm.
- See him stagger back and his hands reach desperately for his face.
- Repeat your mental rehearsal scenario as often as your time allows.
- When the time is up, tell yourself you conquered the attacker and you feel confident as you proceed with your day.

Key Points

- These are just a few of the many things your senses perceive. Be creative and add more.
- If you know where your dream occurred, image that environment so your rehearsal is as real as possible.
- Because you image in real time, you can easily get in 10 reps.

Mini Movements: 10 To 15 Minutes

Let's look at using mini movements to help you overcome your dream issues. Know you can also use mini movements when rehearsing a 2 to 5 "Quick Session" as well as when doing "Deep Meditation." This time, lets use the technique described in "Sitting Meditation 3: Candle or light meditation."

- Find a place to be alone or at least be undisturbed for a few minutes. If this is impossible, sit or stand calmly wherever you might be.
- Then think or whisper your trigger word and feel the first wave of calmness wash over you, from your head to your toes. Think or whisper it two or three times.
- Look at the candle or light for a couple minutes. Just study the light: its brightness or dimness, its flicker, what it illuminates and what it doesn't.

Now you're ready to start your meditation.

- Breathe deeply into your belly and slowly exhale while looking at the candle or light.
- Each time you exhale, think or whisper "calm," "relax," or whatever words connotes to you a quiet, tranquil mind.
- Should your mind wander, don't fret. Just bring it back to the light and your methodical breathing.
- Repeat the inhalation and exhalation procedure for five to eight minutes.

Hold onto this relaxed and calm state as you commence the mini movement mental rehearsal.

- Close your eyes.
- If you normally sit straight in your car seat, do so now. If you slouch, then slouch away.
- Feel the seat on your rear and back, smell the air coming in through the window, taste the mint in your mouth, and hear cars coming and going.
- Turn your head a little to your left and see the figure approaching your door.
- See the door jerked open and physically twitch as if startled for a moment.
- Feel adrenaline surge through your body. Deliberately breathe a little faster.
- Extend your left hand a little and feel your hand grab his reaching arm. Feel and see him try to pull his arm back. Extend yours a little as if being pulled. Then draw your arm back a little as if pulling him toward you. Remember, these are mini movements.
- Move your left foot as if stepping out of your car. Feel it land on the pavement. Drive off with your right foot a little, as if pushing yourself out of the vehicle.
- Hear him curse and threaten.
- Thrust your right palm a little as if striking his face. Though you're moving your arm only two inches, feel your entire body drive your adrenaline-fueled power.
- Feel your palm smash into his nose.
- Hear his loud grunt of pain.

- Physically release your left hand from his forearm. See and feel it release.
- See him stagger back and his hands reach desperately for his face.
- Rehearse whatever outcome applies to you.
- Repeat your mental rehearsal as often as your time allows.
- When the time is up, tell yourself you conquered the attacker and you feel confident as you proceed with your day.

Key Points

- Move your body and limbs no more than a couple of inches, three at the most. Keep the mini in mini movements.
- In your mind, you're twisting completely to see the threat; you're reaching all the way out to grab his arm; you're climbing all the way out of the car; and thrusting your palm-heel strike all the way into the man's face.

Deep Meditation: 15 To 25 Minutes

With the added time to bring on a sense of profound relaxation and calm with meditation, your solution to your dream issue will be more deeply ingrained in your mind. Let's continue with "Sitting Meditation 3: Candle or light meditation."

- Find a place to be alone or at least be undisturbed for a few minutes. If this is impossible, sit or stand calmly wherever you might be.
- Then think or whisper your trigger word and feel the first wave of calmness wash over you, from your head to your toes. Think or whisper it two or three times, and enjoy the sensation of calmness and relaxation.
- Look at the candle or light for a couple of minutes. Just study the light: its brightness or dimness, its flicker, what it illuminates, and what it doesn't.

Now you're ready to start your meditation.

- Breathe deeply into your belly and slowly exhale while looking at the candle or light.

- Each time you exhale, think or whisper "calm," "relax," or whatever words connotes to you a quiet, tranquil mind.
- If your mind drifts off, just bring it back to the light and your breathing.
- Repeat the inhalation and exhalation procedure for five to eight minutes.

Now you're calm and relaxed and receptive to your mental rehearsal.

- Once again you're seated in your vehicle. See, hear, feel, smell, and taste everything in this environment as you did before.
- See the attacker stepping toward your door and feel your adrenaline wash through your muscles.
- Deliberately accelerate your breathing.
- See and hear your door open and feel how it charges your adrenaline even more.
- See the attacker in your mind's eye: sex, age, race, height and weight.
- See his arm reach for you. See and feel your hand reach out to grab it.
- Feel your energy; feel your determination not to be victimized; feel your confidence and courage to stop the attack.
- See and feel yourself step out of the vehicle. Feel your courage and your intent.
- See and feel your palm-heel thrust at the attacker's face. Feel the power and energy behind it.
- Feel your palm smash into his nose.
- See him stagger back.
- Repeat your mental rehearsal as often as your time allows.
- When the time is up, tell yourself you conquered the attacker and you feel confident as you proceed with your day.

Key Points

- The purpose of this rehearsal is to image a positive outcome to a reoccurring dream. As such, I have stopped the rehearsal after you have knocked him away from you. To continue with whatever you would do in a real situation as a martial artist, police officer, or soldier, you would rehearse getting back into

your vehicle and leaving; placing the subject under arrest; or doing whatever procedure is SOP in your military unit
- To be effective, you must take the time to bring on a profound sense of calm and relaxation to imprint imagery into your subconscious.
- The entire scenario should play out in about 10 seconds, thus allowing you to repeat your mental rehearsal multiple times in the 10 minutes or more you've allotted.
- Pause in your mental rehearsal to repeat your keyword three or four times whenever you want to deepen your physical relaxation and mental calm. You can also pause to meditate on the candle or light for a few minutes more. Then continue with your mental rehearsal.

MENTAL REHEARSAL 7: GIVING A PRESENTATION

When you become expert in a given field or you just know more than the next guy, you're likely to be asked to teach it or talk about it in front of others. I've known big burly warriors in the martial arts, police, and military communities who wouldn't hesitate to wade into the murkiest of places. But put them in front of an audience and they fall apart. I'm speaking from personal experience because I fell apart many times.

As the police bureau's gang enforcement spokesperson for white supremacy crimes during the height of the skinhead problem, I gave countless community talks and nearly 200 media interviews. I was never comfortable with the job but I wasn't given a choice. I did, however, have one as to how I prepared. The following was of invaluable help during those years, and still is.

Let's say your superior has just told that he wants you to give a presentation in one hour to a group of people.

Quick Session: 2 To 5 Minutes

- Sit or stand calmly wherever you might be.
- Think or whisper your trigger word and feel the first wave of calmness wash over you, from your head to your toes. Think or whisper it two or three times, and enjoy the sensation of calmness and relaxation.
- Now, inhale slowly and follow your breath as it enters your nose, travels down your throat and chest, and expands your lower belly.
- Exhale slowly as you feel it leave your lower belly, travel up through your chest and throat, and silently exit out your mouth.
- Each time you exhale, think or whisper "calm," "relax," or whatever word connotes to you a quiet, tranquil mind.
- Repeat the inhalation and exhalation procedure two more times. If you can do it four or fives times, do so.

Now you're ready to do a quick mental rehearsal of your presentation.

- See yourself standing at the rear of the room as someone makes your introduction. See the backs of heads, feel the warmth in the room, and feel the butterflies in your gut.
- Hear the sounds of a room: coughs, sniffs, chairs scooting, and whispers.
- Smell the smells of a training facility or a meeting room: perfume, mints, and wet coats.
- See heads turn to look at you when your name is announced.
- Feel yourself walk confidently along the side of the room to the front. Think of the butterflies in your gut as energy to make your presentation dynamic.
- See the many faces as you center yourself on them. Image a pause to collect yourself.
- Hear the beginning of your presentation. Feel your confidence. Feel the sensation of being comfortable in front of the group. Feel the naturalness of your gestures and hear the well-paced clarity of your words.
- Repeat this as many times as you're able.
- When the time is up, tell yourself your rehearsal went well and feel a new confidence as you proceed with your day.

Key Points

- Do not allow a negative thought—I'm so nervous; I sound illiterate; they're whispering about me—to enter your imagery. Think: "I'm polished. I'm confident. I'm in command of myself, the information, and the room."

Mini Movements: 10 To 15 Minutes

Now let's rehearse while making abbreviated movements. Let's use the meditation as described in "Sitting Meditation 5: 8-count breathing.

- Get comfortable wherever you're sitting. Scoot a little this way and that way and wiggle your butt to get your sit-down muscles where you want them.
- Think or whisper your trigger word three times
- Take two or three deep breaths to settle your body and alert your brain as to what you're about to do.

You're now ready to commence the meditation phase.

- Breathe in slowly through your nose to a count of 8: 1, 2, 3, 4, 5, 6, 7, 8.
- Hold it in for a count of 8: 1, 2, 3, 4, 5, 6, 7, 8.
- Exhale out your mouth for a count of 8: 1, 2, 3, 4, 5, 6, 7, 8.
- Hold it for a count of 8: 1, 2, 3, 4, 5, 6, 7, 8.
- Repeat the cycle for as many times as you like to get as mentally calm and physically relaxed as you can.

Now, hold onto this relaxed and calm state as you mentally rehearse using small motions.

- See yourself at the rear of the room and straighten your posture a little. See the backs of heads and turn yours a little as you mentally rehearse scanning the room.
- See and hear another person make your introduction. Physically nod and smile.
- Feel the warmth in the room and feel the butterflies in your gut.
- Hear the sounds of people: coughs, sniffs, chairs scooting, and whispers.

- Smell the smells of a training facility or of a classroom: perfume, mints, wet coats from a rainstorm.
- Move your legs and feet a little as you see and feel yourself walk confidently along the side of the room to the front. Feel your anxiety as dynamic energy.
- See the faces looking at you as you center yourself on the crowd. Turn your head left and right as you look back at them. Make small adjustments as you would in reality—straighten your tie, tuck in your shirt, and so on. Image a short pause to collect yourself.
- Hear the beginning of your presentation. Make small, natural hand gestures and turn your head to the right and left as you mentally rehearse speaking. Feel your confidence. Feel the sensation of being comfortable in front of the group.
- Repeat this as many times as you're able.
- When the time is up, tell yourself your rehearsal went well and feel a new confidence as you proceed with your day.

Key Points

- If you're a pacer, pretend to pace by turning a little to the left and moving your legs a little to duplicate walking. Then turn to your right and do the same thing in that direction. If you use a lot of hand gestures, mimic doing so using small movements.
- If you know what your crowd looks like—students in your class, your academy class, soldiers in your unit—see their faces in your mental rehearsal.

Deep Meditation: 20 To 30 Minutes

Take at least 10 to 15 minutes to get as deeply calm and relaxed as you can. Since you have more time to get receptive to your mental rehearsal, let's use "Sitting Meditation 8: Survey your body; relax your body."

- Sit or stand calmly wherever you might be.
- Think or whisper your trigger word and feel the first wave of calmness wash over you, from your head to your toes. Think or whisper it two or three times and enjoy the sensation of calmness and relaxation.

Now begin the meditation phase.

- Be aware of your head and neck, front, sides, back, and top. See and feel them in your mind—every rise, fall, curve, and bump. If you have a pain anywhere, be aware of it. If you're feeling good in your head and neck, be aware of it.
- Be aware of your shoulders, front, sides, and top. See and feel their shape. If tension is making you hold them high, ignore it for now.
- Be aware of your arms, upper and forearms. See and feel their shape. If you have a pain in one or both of them, be aware of it.
- Be aware of your hands, back, top, and fingers and what they are touching. If they are resting on your knees, feel the cloth of your pants. If they are folded into the classic meditation position—back of your left hand lying in the palm of your right hand, thumbs gently touching—feel the skin-to-skin contact.
- Be aware of your chest, back, and abdomen. See and feel their shape in your mind. If your stomach feels uncomfortably full, or hungry, be aware of it. If your back hurts from sitting, just be aware of it.
- Be aware of your pelvis, front and sides. See and feel its shape.
- Be aware of your rear. See and feel its shape, and feel whatever you're sitting on—the rough hardness of a sandbag; the contours of an ammo box; or the hard discomfort of a wooden chair.
- Be aware of your upper legs. See and feel their shape and how they are positioned. Be aware of whatever the backs of your legs are touching. Be aware of any pain in your legs.
- Be aware of your calves. See and feel their shape in your mind.
- Be aware of your feet. See and feel their shape. Feel whatever is on your feet. If you're barefoot, feel whatever they are resting upon.

You just did the awareness stage. Now proceed to more deeply relax your body.

- Be aware of your head and neck, front, sides, back, and top as you inhale. Each time you exhale, see and feel your muscles, tendons, and skin melting over your skull into deep relaxation. Repeat two, three, or four times.
- Be aware of your shoulders, front, sides, and top as you inhale.

As you exhale, feel them sink and grow heavy. Repeat until the area is completely relaxed.
- Be aware of your arms, upper and forearms, as you inhale. Each time you exhale, feel them become profoundly heavy and relaxed. Repeat two, three, or four times.
- Be aware of your hands, back, top, and fingers as you inhale. As you exhale, see and feel them become so light they could float upward. Repeat two, three, or four times.
- Be aware of your chest, back, and abdomen as you inhale. Each time you exhale, see and feel them sink and relax. If you're sitting with your spine straight, relax into it without allowing it to slump. Repeat two, three, or four times.
- Be aware of your pelvis, front and sides as you inhale. Each time you exhale, see and feel it grow heavier and heavier. Repeat two, three, or four times.
- Be aware of your butt as you inhale. Each time you exhale, feel it become heavy as it sinks into whatever it's sitting on. Repeat two, three, or four times.
- Be aware of your upper legs as you inhale. Each time you exhale, see and feel them become heavy and sink into whatever they are touching. Repeat two, three, or four times.
- Be aware of your calves as you inhale. Each time you exhale, see and feel them relax and become heavy. Repeat two, three, or four times.
- Be aware of your feet as you inhale. Each time you exhale, see and feel them grow heavy as they sink into whatever they are touching. Repeat two, three, or four times.

Hold onto this relaxed and calm state as you mentally rehearse.

- See and hear another person make your introduction.
- See yourself at the rear of the room and, as you do, straighten your posture a little. See the backs of heads.
- Feel the warmth in the room and feel the butterflies in your gut.
- Hear the sounds of people: coughs, sniffs, chairs scooting, and whispers.
- Smell the smells of a training facility or of a meeting: perfume, mints, and wet coats.
- See and feel yourself walk confidently along the side of the room to the front. Feel your anxiety as dynamic energy.

- See faces looking at you as you center yourself on the crowd. Image a short pause to collect yourself.
- Hear the beginning of your presentation. See yourself make small, natural hand gestures and make eye contact with the crowd. Feel your confidence.
- Feel the sensation of being comfortable in front of the group.
- Repeat this as many times as you're able.
- When the time is up, tell yourself your rehearsal went well and that you feel a new confidence as you proceed with your day.

Key Points

- If you know your audience, bring additional detail into your mental rehearsal. Be an actor for a few minutes and play your part over and over. The more real you can make it, the greater the benefit to you.

A Gimmick I Found Useful

Johnny Carson was still hosting *The Tonight Show* when I was working in the gang unit and doing so many television, radio, and newspaper interviews. To my mind, he was the consummate example of someone who functioned well in front of an audience. In his case, several million people a night.

I never tried to imitate him but I often mentally rehearsed seeing myself just as confident, smooth, dignified, and unruffled as Carson. As you might recall, when he did goof up something, he never let it affect him. Imaging those attributes, not as Carson but as myself, played an important role in many of my pre-presentation mental rehearsal sessions.

Who might yours be? Brian Williams is good. So are many candidates for office since they have been groomed to function well in front of a crowd.

CHAPTER 10

MENTAL REHEASAL WITHOUT MEDITATION

As reiterated throughout this guide, meditating before practicing mental rehearsal produces a suggestible mind that is receptive to your input. However, there is evidence that shows you can get some results without meditating first.

Weight Training

In one study published in the *Journal of Conditioning Research,* (2010), weight trainees who imaged doing leg presses were able to lift more weight and do more repetitions than those who didn't.

Here is one way to do that with dumbbell curls. Instead of chatting with friends or posing in the wall mirror during your 60-second rest between sets, mentally rehearse as follows:

- If you've been curling, say, 35-pound dumbbells, see yourself pick up the 40-pounders.
- See and feel the motion of your arms curling the dumbbells.
- Feel an extraordinary burst of strength and energy in your biceps.
- See your arms the way you want them to be—big, shapely, full of power and strength—as you rehearse the curling motion.

You might not be able to curl those 40s on your next set, but keep mentally rehearsing it and you will get there sooner than if you hadn't imaged at all during your rest periods.

Lose Fat

A study published in the *Journal of Behavioral Medicine*, 2011, reported that people who imaged themselves with the slimmer physique they wanted burned more calories than those who didn't practice imagery.

The best time to do this is as you prepare to exercise. Image the following as you put on your martial arts training clothes, change into to your military PT clothes, or slip on your shorts and T-shirt for a run after your patrol shift:

- See clearly in your mind the physique you want.
- See and feel yourself leaner, stronger, and harder.
- See it and feel as you dress or in any other way prepare to train.

Train When You're Too Tired

I've done this a thousand times, probably more. I'm exhausted, beat, trashed, pooped, or just plain don't want to train. All I want to do is sprawl on the sofa and work my thumb muscles on the TV remote. But that darn discipline kicks in and I drag my sorry self off to change into my karate pants and T-shirt. In the three or four minutes it takes to change, a powerful transformation takes place. Here is how you can do it on those days you've been road hard and put away wet.

- As you change, feel new energy course through your body.
- See one small aspect of the training to come: sidekicks on the heavy bag; clearing the first obstacle on a mile-long running course; or practicing prone handcuffing. Feel the energy needed for the task. Feel it course through you.
- See and feel these things all the while you change into the clothing you use specifically for training.

Post-it Notes

Yup, those little sticky papers can help you shoot better, fight better, kick in a door better, and improve nearly everything else you do in your warrior life. How? It's all about the power of words and how they trigger your mind.

Let's say you have one of the following issues:

A. You consistently pull to the right at the firing range.
B. You get nervous when talking before a group.
C. You fail to watch the student-suspect's hands when practicing scenarios.
D. You fail to watch all 360 degrees when on a mission.

Maybe you have trouble remembering certain elements under stress or maybe you simply have a bad memory. The solution: Post-it Notes.

Okay, that's really not THE solution but it will help by keeping the fix—the mental image—in the forefront of your mind.

Begin by choosing one or two words, maybe a sentence that works for you and your issue. It doesn't matter what the word(s) are as long as it works for you. Maybe it's something your instructor or sergeant said. Maybe it's a buzzword or term you've heard that works in your mind. It doesn't matter *as long as it works for you.*

Referring to the above problems, here are some examples. Got better ones? Use 'em.

A. "Grip" "Breathe" "Relax"
B. "Slow Down" "Pause" [Write down the name of someone to emulate]
C. "Watch Hands" "Hands" "Watch"
D. "360" "Watch My Six" "Alert"

Put the Post-it on your bathroom mirror, inside your locker door, car dash, beer mug, and anywhere else where you can see it several times a day. When you see the Post-It and your word(s), let the meaning form an image in your mind. Reflect for a moment longer and then continue about your business.

You will like the results.

→ **BONUS** ←

CHAPTER 11

MENTAL REHEARSAL FOR SCHOOL TEACHERS

In the few months it took to write this small book, there were several active shooter incidents at schools and one mass stabbing. One of the schools was in my city, about three miles away. There were also random shootings at workplaces and a military base. In the event some warrior readers have spouses, relatives, or friends working in the school system—I have three—I want to give you one mental rehearsal method for teachers and administrators. Please pass this on to them. This is taken in part from my book, *Surviving a School Shooting*.

School teachers now have to be concerned about irate parents and students who choose to settle their personal issues with firearms or a blade. To make matters worse, too many are in denial that such a thing could ever happen at their school. Well, there were also deniers in every school where it's occurred in the last 15 to 20 years.

But it happened, anyway.

Still, there are too many who won't take proactive measures, such as running drills or even discussing it. Fortunately, I hear from people who do think about it, worry about it, try to be proactive in their schools, and personally practice mental rehearsal.

The following exercise is one small but effective proactive step teachers and administrators can do.

This can be done in the home, teachers lounge, private car, and in your classroom when you have a prep period. As mentioned throughout this book, you're encouraged to calm your mind first through meditation so it's more receptive to your mental rehearsal. Please choose one of the aforementioned methods.

For our purposes here, let's go straight to the mental rehearsal. Let's make the setting a classroom.

- See your environment: students, chalkboards, chairs, desks, and wall maps. See where you are in the room.
- Smell the usual odors associated with the classroom: chalk, glue, and old books.
- Hear running steps from out in the hall followed by screams and the sound of two gunshots. Hear the students around you shout and cry out in fear. Hear their chairs scoot on the floor.
- Smell and taste gun smoke wafting through the open door.
- Feel your quickening heart beat.

If you feel anxious at this point in your mental rehearsal, take a moment to say or whisper your trigger word. Then continue.

- Hear screams and more shots from out in the hall. See and hear your students beginning to panic.
- See yourself rush toward the door as you gesture for the students to move to the rear of the classroom.
- Feel your hand touch the door, and push it quickly but quietly shut. Feel your fingers grasp the door lock and turn it. See and feel your hands reach for the light switch and switch it off. Feel your hand pull down the curtain.
- The last thing you see is the shooter at the other end of the hall walking around the corner, a rifle in each hand.
- Feel your pulse and breathing quicken.

If you feel anxious at this point in your mental rehearsal, take a moment to say or whisper your trigger word. Tell yourself you will remain calm and in control right now, as well as in a real event. Then continue.

- See yourself gesturing for two big kids to help push your desk over to block the door, even if it opens outward into the hall. (Seeing the barricade might discourage the shooter or slow him down.)
- See yourself waving your hands to the students to get their

attention. See yourself put a finger to your lips for them to be quiet. See yourself pantomime holding a rifle and see yourself point toward the door so they know what you mean.
- See yourself move quickly toward the back of the classroom with the others and gesture for everyone to get down on the floor.
- Hear another shot from out in the hall. Hear more running footsteps. Hear a scream.

If at this point you feel anxious in your mental rehearsal, take a moment to say or whisper your trigger word. Tell yourself you will remain calm and in control right now and in a real event. Then continue.

- Feel yourself hug the floor and hold the hand of the student next to you.
- Hear yourself whisper for everyone to stay down and remain quiet.
- See frightened faces looking at you.
- See and feel your hand reach out to comfort a student who is starting to lose control.
- Hear the doorknob rattle and hear students whimper.
- Take a deep breath to retain your control.
- See the doorknob stop turning.
- Hear footsteps outside the door walking away.

Key Points

- Remain with the basic mental rehearsal for a few sessions before adding other elements, such as grabbing a weapon common to your classroom—scissors, stapler, chair, heavy book, laptop, and anything else that could hurt and stop a threat. If there is a window, see yourself ushering students through it.

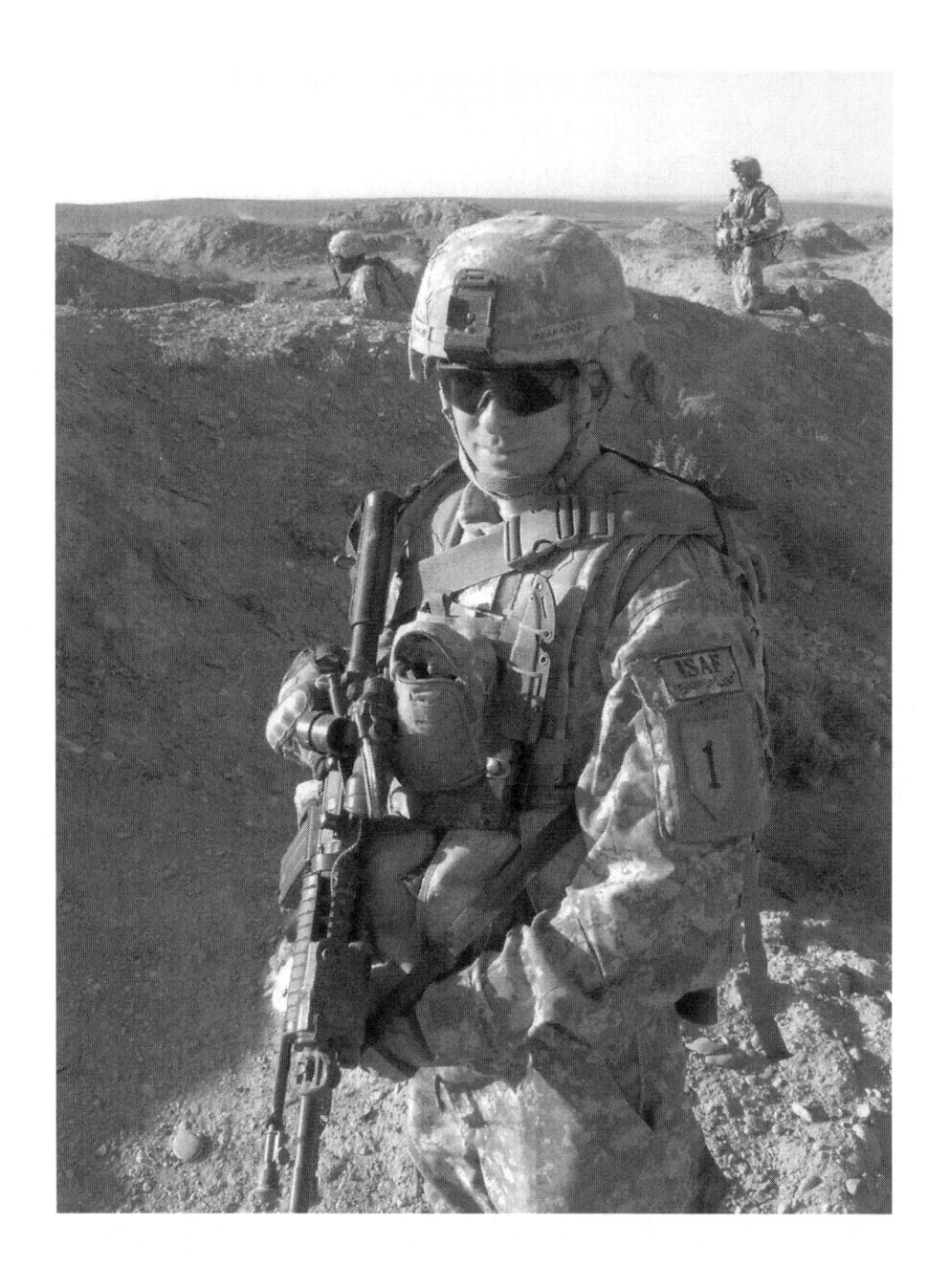

CONCLUSION

In the event you're still doubtful about the power of mental rehearsal, know that it works even if you don't believe in it. This is because it's not about a belief system or faith. Mental rehearsal works because the images you create—complete with the involvement of your five senses—are believed in your mind to be as real as your physical kick/punch drill, handcuffing technique, or an all-out gunfight.

Your ultra clear mental images are often said to be the language of your body, the only one it recognizes instantly. To say it another way, your body and mind don't differentiate between what you conjure in your mental rehearsal and what you see and do in reality.

In the very near future, mental rehearsal will be a natural part of every warrior's training regimen, as natural as shooting, grappling, jumping out of a plane, and running laps. Why wait for the future? Others aren't.

Stay safe out there ~ Loren W. Christensen

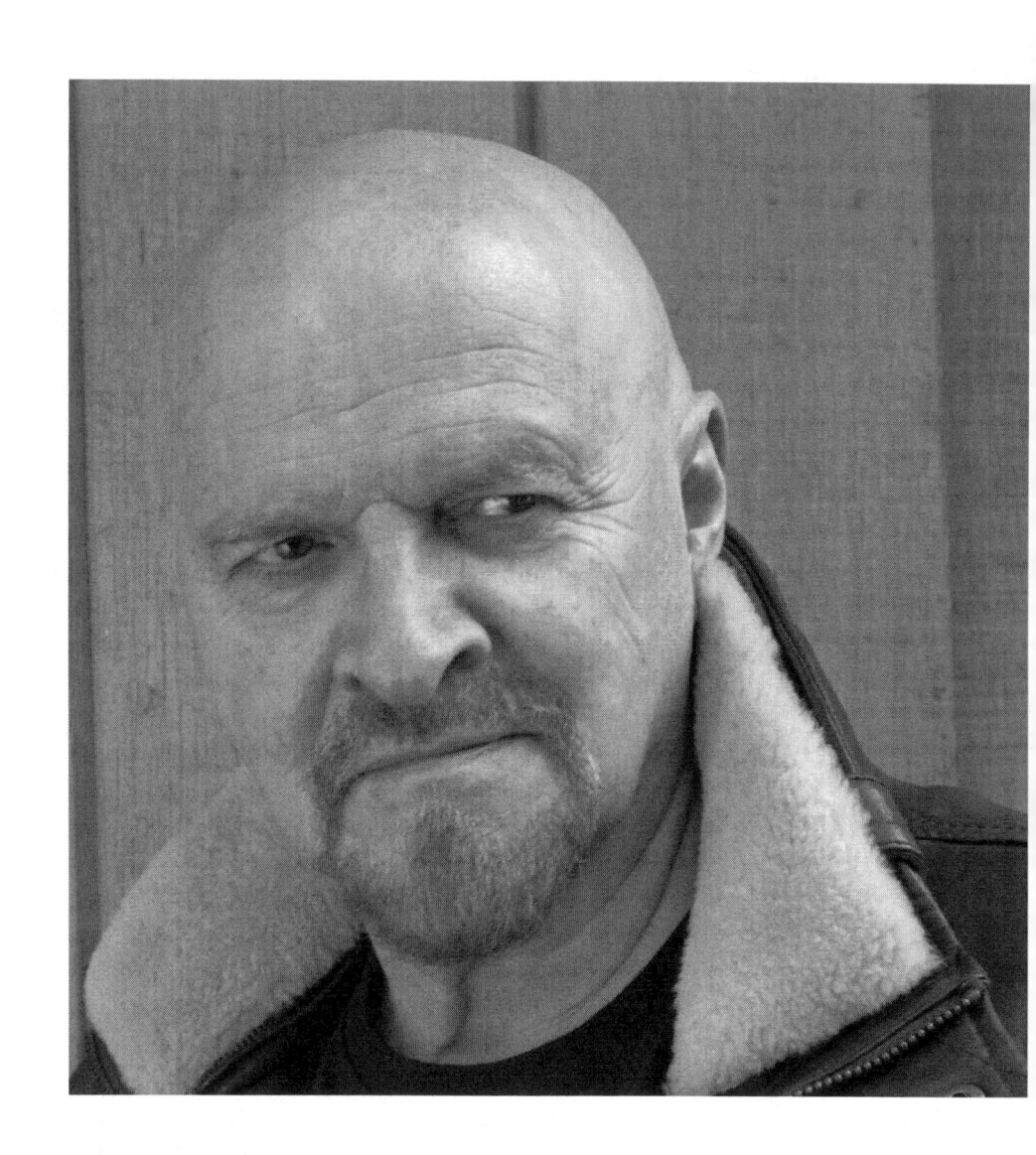

ABOUT THE AUTHOR

Loren W. Christensen is a Vietnam veteran and retired police officer with 29 years of law enforcement experience.

As a martial arts student and teacher since 1965, he has earned a total of 11 black belts in three arts and was inducted into the Masters Hall of Fame in 2011. He has starred in seven instructional martial arts DVDs.

As a writer, Loren has worked with five publishers, penning 46 nonfiction books on a variety of subjects, a thriller fiction series called *Dukkha*, and dozens of magazine articles.

Loren has been a student of meditation since 1990.

Loren W. Christensen DVDs

Solo Training
Fighting Dirty
Speed Training
Masters and Styles
Vital Targets
The Brutal Art of Ripping, and Pressing Vital Targets
Restraint and Control Strategies

Made in the USA
Middletown, DE
01 September 2015